MW01632050

Achieving Mid-life Vitality

Hormone Balance and Beyond

Karen Sun, M.D.

with Gino Tutera, M.D.

Sunshine Publications

PUBLISHER'S NOTE:

AN IMPORTANT CAUTION TO OUR READERS:

This book is not a medical manual and cannot take the place of personalized medical advice and treatment from a qualified physician. The reader should regularly consult a physician in matters relating to his or her health, particularly with respect to any symptoms that may require diagnosis or treatment. Although certain medical procedures and medical professionals are mentioned in this book, no endorsement, warranty or guarantee by the author is intended. Every attempt has been made to ensure that the information contained in this book is current, however, due to the fact that research is ongoing, some of the material may be invalidated by new findings. The author and publisher cannot guarantee that the information and advice in this book are safe and proper for every reader. For that reason, this book is sold without warranties or guarantees of any kind, expressed or implied, and the author and publisher disclaim any liability, loss or damage caused by the contents. If you do not wish to be bound by these cautions and conditions, you may return your copy to the publisher for a full refund.

Printed in the United States of America

Sun, Karen with Tutera, Gino
Achieving Mid-life Vitality: Hormone Balance and Beyond

ISBN: 978-1-61539-185-1
LCCN: 2009903100

Cover design: Christy Salinas

Published by:
Sunshine Publications
4 Hughes - Ste 150
Irvine, CA 92618

Dedication

I dedicate this book to my parents, Ching Mai Sun and Han Chin Sun. Without them I would not be who I am today. They both passed away in 2008 and they will always be in my memory for the love and support they gave me.

This book is also dedicated to all my patients who I learned from their experience about healthy aging, disease prevention, and hormone balance.

TABLE OF CONTENTS

Acknowledgements

I wish to express my gratitude to Dr. Gino Tutera for sharing his knowledge and wisdom on how to treat men and women with hormone pellets. His expertise has allowed me to help my patients to a much greater extent than other routes of hormone therapy. He also coauthored with me on the chapters regarding hormone treatment.

I thank my editors Melissa Wells and Miguel Cervantes, for their encouragement and hard work to bring this project to completion. Melissa Wells also did all the interviews of my patients and wrote their stories, I appreciate her wonderful work.

Many thanks go to Dr. Ling Huang, L.Ac. for her contribution in writing of the acupuncture chapter. Gary Groves, M.D. helped to edit the manuscript and gave me many of his precious opinions and I truly appreciate his help.

I thank my office staff, Rose Riojas, Yvonne Wang, Crystal Martinez, Rose Lin, and Amy Huang for their dedication and support. I thank Sebastian Cervantes for the research hours he contributed. I thank Steve and Helen Kay for their friendship and spiritual guidance.

Lastly, my heartfelt thanks go to my husband for his loving support throughout this process and doing more than his share of taking care of our son, Michael, allowing me the time to write.

— *Karen Sun, M.D.*

Introduction

Are you a middle-aged woman suffering from hot flashes, insomnia, moodiness, and weight gain?

Are you a middle-aged man suffering from declining energy, memory, and libido?

Are you curious about the pros and cons of hormone replacement therapy, and what form is the safest and most effective?

Are you aware of the toxins in our environment and the ways to help your body detoxify?

Do you want to reduce your stress levels, and experience more peace and joy in your life?

Do you want to know how to eat in order to reduce inflammation, indigestion, and lose weight?

Do you want to prevent heart disease, stroke, cancer, and Alzheimer's disease?

Do you want to slow the aging process down and regain the vitality you once had?

If you answered "*yes*" to any one of the questions above, this book is for you, as it has been written for people who want to take charge of their own health and healing. Knowledge is power, and the more you know about your body and the many factors that influence your health and well-being, the more empowered you will be to make informed decisions that will improve the quality of your entire life.

The quest to achieve a true and lasting healing of the body and to balance those needs with those of the mind and spirit is a goal that many share, and one that I have pursued throughout my professional career. The search has been exhaustive, with gains and setbacks along the way. What I have discovered are the keys to balancing the fundamental cornerstones of our physical, mental, and emotional health, well into mature adulthood. This journey has enabled thousands of patients regain their vitality, and enjoy healthy and active lives at any age. In this book I would like to share these discoveries with you.

My Story

Throughout my life, I have always been accustomed to living in high gear. Like most of the women I see in my practice, I have had to juggle multiple roles. Long hours of work and study, worrying about the health of my patients, running the day-to-day business of a private practice, taking care of my elderly parents and trying to be a good mother and wife at the same time—the challenges have been never ending. Like most women, I have been the last person that I have had time for.

My health was not great in my younger years. I developed scoliosis early in life and suffered through many years of neck and back pain. My stomach became extremely sensitive and reacted to many types of foods with abdominal pain and bloating. My energy fluctuated throughout the day, even after a full night's rest. I also experienced heavy menstrual bleeding and cramps. Yet, despite the clear warning signs that my body was sending—I continued to press on, convinced that the rewards of a fast-paced lifestyle were more than worth the effort.

By the time I entered menopause in my early 50s, things had changed. I had hot flashes that woke me up at night, and poor sleep that lead to a decline in memory and energy. Handling daily tasks became more difficult. My skin became dryer, I had more aches and pains and nothing seemed to interest me any more. I became frustrated, to say the least. My ob-gyn suggested antidepressants for the hot flashes and to help improve my sleep. Being an internist, I knew better than to risk the potential side effects of these drugs. I did not like the idea of taking birth control pills or oral estrogen, since their side effects are well documented. My desire to avoid the use of heavy-duty drugs led me to try a more benign approach that included natural hormones like progesterone creams and estradiol patches, knowing they would attempt to mimic the hormones my body once produced. Due to my hectic schedule, however, I would often forget to reapply the creams or replace the patches, only to wake up with night sweats the next night. Plus, I was still tired throughout the day and not feeling well overall.

The answer came one day during a routine consultation when one of my patients introduced me to a book titled *You Don't Have to Live with It*, by Gino Tutera M.D. My patient explained to me that Dr. Tutera was experiencing groundbreaking success in treating men and women experiencing a variety of conditions associated with mid-life hormonal changes using bio-identical hormone pellets. I initially reacted with skepticism. Many questions came to mind, such as: "What is this? Why have I not heard about this? Is it dangerous?" I had many reservations about reading Dr. Tutera's book, not to mention my packed patient schedule. Yet, by this time the undesirable symptoms associated with my transition into menopause, coupled with the aches and pains accumulated from my overworked lifestyle, had become a constant ordeal. My experience with hormone creams and patches had already opened my eyes to the possibilities of hormone therapy, so I set aside my doubts and read the book. Interestingly, I found that the information it contained made a great deal of sense. Dr. Tutera's approach was straightforward and based on solid medical research.

Encouraged by this, I made the decision to attend Dr. Tutera's training seminar in Scottsdale, Arizona; where I learned how to implant bio-identical hormone pellets just under the skin to treat hormonal imbalances. Immediately after the training, I treated a few of my patients with the pellets who were not responding to hormone creams and patches. The results were immediate and startling. Every one of these patients experienced a dramatic improvement! So, I decided to begin treatment with bio-identical hormone pellets on myself. It turned out to be one of the best decisions I have ever made. My symptoms disappeared! As a matter of fact, the third morning after the pellet implant, I slept like a baby, arose early in the morning refreshed, and went for a vigorous jog. I felt energetic and happy for the first time in a long time.

From then on, I introduced the pellets to some of my patients who had been using hormone creams with questionable results. Their improvement was immediate and noticeable as well. Symptoms that responded only mildly to hormone creams disappeared completely once the pellets were implanted. As a result of the wonderful improvement in my patient's health, the news began to spread. As everyone knows, a good secret can be hard to keep, especially when the benefits are so readily apparent both inside and out, as they clearly are with bio-identical hormone therapy. A steady stream of patient referrals began to inundate my appointment lists. Many of these new patients had to drive hours to get to my practice and quite a few traveled from out of state. Many were desparate to find relief and had heard of my success treating patients with bio-identical hormone pellet therapy after having exhausted just about every other means of conventional and alternative treatments. So beneficial were these powerful little pellets, and so rapid was the spread of their praise that within a span of three years my practice had grown to more than 1,000 patients who were benefiting from bio-identical hormone pellet therapy, a powerful testimony to its effectiveness.

Gradually, men began showing up in my office too. Usually their wife or girlfriend had received treatment from me first. After witnessing the dramatic change their partner experienced, particularly in their improved libido, they became eager to try this treatment for themselves. Today, it is no longer a secret that men can benefit from pellet therapy. Especially, professional men with stressful jobs, who upon reaching middle-age find themselves becoming more irritable and short tempered, and feel that they are losing their energy, mental sharpness and vitality. Many of the men who come to see me have heard of testosterone shots, but they are unaware of the many advantages in safety and efficacy that bio-identical testosterone pellets offer. Once they experience the remarkable benefits of treatment, they are quick to embrace this approach as well.

There is no doubt that pellet therapy can be a powerful and life-altering experience for many people. In my quest to fulfill my patients' desires for optimal health, I came to realize that hormones are only one part of the solution. I continued my study and research, and attended seminars offered by organizations such as The American College of Advanced Medicine (ACAM) and The Institute of Functional medicine (IFM). From those seminars I learned how to treat the root causes of disease, not just the symptoms. I also learned how to combine conventional treatment methods with alternative approaches to produce therapies that work.

During the course of my practice in medicine, I also came to realize that treating the body is not enough. The body also houses our mind and spirit. Unless the mind and spirit are at ease, the body will become dis–eased. In 2008, both my parents passed away. It was a hard year for me emotionally, and their passing proved to be a major turning point in my life. I experienced a spiritual awakening that helped me to see that everything in this world is temporary and illusory, and that it is never worthwhile to let anger or hate become our sole point of focus. Love is what is truly important, along with forgiveness and living in the present. We all have important missions to fulfill in our lives, and I believe we are here to learn lessons, enjoy life, and help other people as much as we can.

My Observations

Official statistics estimate that the majority of women today suffer from a variety of unpleasant conditions during their menopausal years. While a small portion of women are able to make the transition through menopause with little to no difficulty, a roughly equal to greater number remain on the opposite end of the spectrum, suffering intensely from a variety of uncomfortable and in many cases debilitating health issues that dramatically affect their quality of life.

It has been my observation that most patients suffering from severe menopausal symptoms also have adrenal fatigue. This condition occurs when the adrenal glands function below their optimal levels and is usually caused by chronic stress. Before menopause, the adrenal glands contribute approximately 30 percent of the sex hormone production and more than 70 percent after menopause. When the adrenal glands become burned out, they are not able to produce the sex hormones a woman's body requires after menopause. I fit into this category as an overworked career woman. Patients with mild cases of adrenal fatigue respond wonderfully to pellet therapy, as it helps them to sleep better and increases their energy level. Patients in moderate to severe stages of adrenal fatigue need additional treatment, such as adrenal support products and vitamin supplements. Most importantly, however, they need to incorporate major lifestyle changes to reduce the stressors in their lives.

Thyroid is another hormone that plays a vital role in energy production. I have seen many patients with thyroid function tests in the lower range of normal who nonetheless have all the symptoms of hypothyroidism. These people gain weight easily, and have a hard time losing weight. This type of subclinical (undiagnosed) hypothyroidism is very common, especially in menopausal women, and a low dosage of thyroid medication helps provide health improvement.

I have also observed that certain patients have an adverse response to pellet therapy. In these cases, it is likely that their hormone receptors are altered due to the effects of the accumulation of toxins in their bodies. Usually, they also suffer from other problems such as multiple chemical sensitivities, leaky gut syndrome, autoimmune diseases, or mercury toxicity. This group of patients is more difficult to treat. Often, a detoxification program is a necessary first step in treatment. Also, due to their increased sensitivity their pellet dosages need to be carefully adjusted.

My Theory

Women are much more stressed now, due to juggling family lives and careers, not to mention taking care of everyone else's needs rather than their own. By the time menopause comes around, the adrenal glands are burned out when the ovaries have quit working. The adrenal glands are supposed to take over the production of sex hormones in women after menopause. But, due to adrenal fatigue, more and more women are experiencing very uncomfortable and sometimes debilitating menopausal symptoms.

Men, on the other hand, are not much better off. Chronic stress also causes adrenal fatigue, which reduces the testosterone production from the adrenal glands. Andropause, the term coined to describe male menopause, develops more gradually but earlier, with their own debilitating symptoms like low libido, fatigue, weight gain, mental fog, and cardiovascular diseases.

Stress management has become "Survival 101." Without changing our thoughts and value systems, we will not be able to gain control over the continual firing line of stressors we are exposed to in today's world. Stress coping skills such as meditation, creative visualization, and relaxation exercises are important survival tools as we grow older.

We also live in a very toxic world, tremendously more so than previous generations. By the time we reach middle-age, we have accumulated enough toxins in our body to seriously interrupt our hormone systems. The damage is much more pervasive as the body's toxic load interferes with our brain functions, and causes inflammation in the body that can lead to neurodegenerative diseases, cardiovascular diseases, and cancer. Because of each person's unique genetics, the body's detoxification capacities differ. This is why some people, but not all people, suffer from diseases such as chronic fatigue syndrome, fibromyalgia, breast cancer, and multiple chemical sensitivities. If we do not pay attention to the toxins in and around us, we run the risk of becoming victims of these diseases sooner or later.

To regain the vitality we once had, hormone balance is the first essential step. Stress management and detoxification are the next steps, which involves lifestyle modification, developing stress coping skills, along with optimal nutrition and taking supplements that help the body detoxify. The last and most important step is achieving emotional and spiritual health.

How to Use This Book

The information is presented in a simple and straightforward manner to provide everyone with the opportunity to improve their own health. It is divided into four major sections:

I. Understanding the disease process and aging.
II. The ultimate hormone replacement therapy.
III. The importance of the mind-body connection.
IV. A comprehensive program to prevent the diseases associated with aging and to achieve mid-life vitality.

Jump-start your health and well-being program right away by turning to any chapter that is relevant to your current health concerns. These chapters include special topics of focus such as:

Breast Cancer Prevention	see page	57
Make Sleep a Priority	see page	264
Anti-inflammation Diet	see page	132
Healthy Aging Diet	see page	134
Toxin Avoidance	see pages	166-167
Basic Detoxification	see pages	174-175
Meditation	see pages	209-210
Steps for Creative Visualization and Positive Affirmations	see pages	211-212

It is my sincere hope that the information contained in this book helps you prevent disease, achieve optimal health, and slow down the aging process, while experiencing peak physical vitality, mental clarity, and emotional well-being throughout your lifetime.

To your health and vitality!

Achieving Mid-life Vitality

Hormone Balance and Beyond

Part I:

Understanding the Disease Process and Aging

CHAPTER 1

How Diseases Start

Modern medicine has done great things to improve the quality of our lives. Over the course of the last century, its ability to understand disease has made incredible progress. Significant advances in key areas of medical research and technology have enabled physicians to employ increasingly sophisticated techniques in the treatment of illnesses. For example, impressive innovations in the field of diagnostic technology including imaging methods like computed tomography (CT) and magnetic resonance imaging (MRI)—allow physicians to accurately and rapidly diagnose diseases in patients, and help them to spot potential problems ahead of time. Major advances have been made in treating cancer, heart disease, and other acute and chronic diseases with surgery and medications.

But modern medicine also has major shortcomings. It focuses more on treating diseases rather than preventing them from occurring in the first place. With modern medicine's emphasis on medication or surgery as its main tools, it is much better suited to treat acute illnesses, rather than chronic conditions. Indeed, there are times when people will need antibiotics to knock out infections or pain killers to alleviate headaches. But for chronic illnesses such as hypertension, diabetes or arthritis, treatment by medication alone solves only part of the problem. Consideration must also be given to proper nutrition and necessary lifestyle practices, such as maintaining proper weight, getting regular exercise, managing stress, and avoiding tobacco as well as excessive use of alcohol.

Another concern about modern medicine is that it divides diseases into separate systems instead of viewing the body's systems as closely interrelated. Specialists and subspecialists for everything worsen this fragmented perspective. While focusing on a single system has helped doctors to better understand the disease process within each system of the body, this narrow view often ignores the fact that a symptom can have complex causative factors involving many body systems. A headache, for example, can be brought on by emotional issues, food sensitivities, hypertension, hormonal imbalance, recurring stress, allergies, or several of these factors combined. So, if a doctor were to treat a patient complaining of a headache with pain medication the symptoms might well subside for the time being, but the underlying or root cause of the headache will not have been addressed. As a result, the headaches might continue to come back and neither patient nor physician will be aware of the deeper, persistent problems at work. Furthermore, the long-term use of pain medication carries with it the potential for dangerous side effects such as stomach ulcers, kidney or liver damage, and even addiction, all of which contribute to more health problems.

Symptoms are like the leaves on a tree. If you trim the leaves but leave the roots intact, the leaves are guaranteed to return. It is important to look for and treat the root causes of disease so that patients can achieve a deep and truly effective healing—one that helps to ensure a lasting return to good health.

Root Causes of Diseases

We all inherit different sets of genes from our parents, which can make us prone to certain illnesses. This does not necessarily mean that we will get these diseases. A lifestyle burdened by unhealthy habits, however, can make these diseases much more likely to affect us. If adult-onset (Type II) diabetes runs in your family for example, and if you live a sedentary lifestyle that includes poor diet and lack of exercise, then the likelihood that you will develop diabetes will dramatically increase.

But, if you watch your diet, exercise regularly, maintain proper weight and manage stressors well, then your likelihood of developing diabetes will be greatly reduced.

Lifestyle is a major factor that has the power to aggravate or prevent many diseases. This is true not only for genetically inherited diseases, but for many other diseases as well.

Four Factors that Influence Health

The following four factors play a major role in determining an individual's overall health and well-being. Maintaining a healthy balance between these factors is especially important for individuals whose bodies have begun to curtail or cease production of the vital hormones that allow us to cope with stressors and imbalances in our lifestyles.

1. **Nutrition:** We are what we eat. Eating a balanced diet helps to build a strong body. The GI (gastrointestinal) tract plays an important role in our health, as its function is to digest and absorb nutrients. It also serves as a first line of defense to prevent toxins, bacteria, or large food molecules from entering our bodies.

2. **Mental processes:** We are what we think. The mind is the arbiter of our thoughts and emotions. Positive thoughts lead to a mental state where feelings of peace, calm, and happiness flow naturally, while a consistently negative outlook on life can make one far more vulnerable to stress, anxiety, depression and fear.

3. **Toxins:** We live in a world full of toxins. Our body also produces free radicals through chemical reactions that are continually occurring. If we are exposed to more toxins than our body's detoxification system can handle, or more free radicals than our antioxidants can neutralize, then toxins start to accumulate, leading to damage.

   Toxins cause inflammation, which contributes to degenerative diseases like arthritis, atherosclerosis, or Alzheimer's disease. Toxins also cause DNA mutations that lead to cancer. Additionally, toxins weaken our immune system, which leads to allergies, infections, and autoimmune diseases.

4. **Hormones:** Our body's hormones are the chemical messengers that govern how cells, tissues and organs communicate with each other. There are many different kinds of

hormones that are typically categorized as either major or minor, depending upon the role they play and the amount of influence they exert upon our body's functions. Certain major hormones such as thyroid and adrenal hormones are so critical to our health that without them we run the risk of disease and death. Without minor hormones like estrogen and testosterone, our body's ability to function optimally is critically impaired.

If our hormones are in plentiful supply, balanced, and working together then our body will have the tools it needs to function optimally. We will look our best, feel our best, and enjoy the benefits of renewed energy and vitality as the aging process dramatically slows down.

In addition to exerting a fundamental influence on our health, all four of these factors are closely interrelated. If you suffer from hormonal imbalance, for instance, you may feel tired, depressed, moody or anxious. If you are stressed, you may not eat the best foods, exercise properly or sleep well. If you are exposed to certain toxins that disrupt your thyroid hormones, you will gain weight and feel sluggish, even if you eat well and exercise regularly.

Activating Your Healing Systems

Having a healthy body is important, but the extent that we can fully embrace optimum health is largely determined by our mental and emotional state as well. A healthy body depends on an active, alert mind, which in turn draws support from our balanced emotions and strength of spirit. This vital balance of mind, body and spirit is the cornerstone of our health and well-being. In order to get well and stay well, we need to manage all the root factors of disease in order to promote our own internal healing systems.

The answer to the wide array of issues facing our health in the world today lies in a multifaceted approach that takes each aspect of our individuality into account. If we improve our nutritional habits, make exercise a priority, foster emotional well-being, reduce the stressors in our lives, balance our hormones, maintain proper weight, avoid tobacco and excessive alcohol, and use supplements to aid in the prevention of disease we will have taken crucial and empowering steps toward the goal of living long, healthy, and happy lives.

CHAPTER 2

Theories of Aging

Aging is the only fatal affliction that all of us share.

—Leonard Hayflick, Ph.D.

A few years ago I attended my 30-year high school reunion. Since I had gone to an all-girls' school, I saw a room full of middle-aged women. They had familiar faces and voices, yet were very different from what I remembered during our teenage years. Some had gained a lot of weight and others had gray hair. But even those who had not gained weight or grayed still had different faces, due to sagging skin that had fine wrinkles or lost its elasticity. I felt that I was in a time machine tunnel that had moved way too fast!

While aging is an inevitable fact of life, there are many things we can do to slow down the process. Before we discuss these approaches, let us take a moment to go behind the scenes of the aging process and examine its primary causes. Alongside the many advances in the study of medicine today have come several promising theories that help to explain the fundamental causes of aging.

Gene Control Theory and Telomeres

Each time a cell in the body duplicates, it creates entirely new structures of DNA called chromosomes. Telomeres (derived from the Greek telos, or end, and meres, or part) are small fragments of DNA that form the protective ends of chromosomes. The telomeres protect a cell's chromosomes from fusing with each other or rearranging. Each time the chromosomes duplicate, the telomeres get a little shorter, and after their structures shrink to a certain size, cell division stops. At this point, no additional new cells can be made.

One abnormality of this cell duplication process is a genetic disorder called progeria, an accelerated aging disease. Progeria is an extremely rare condition. An individual affected by progeria looks like a miniature elderly person and typically do not live past 10 years of age. Children afflicted with this condition develop the diseases associated with aging, such as arthritis, osteoporosis, and heart attacks.

Rare diseases like progeria have helped to focus increased attention on the issues of aging and longevity, and their link to our genes. Studies have observed that certain species of animals have programmed life spans. For human beings, the genetic potential for longevity has been estimated at about 120 years. Most people, however, never meet this potential due to premature aging, or because they are genetically susceptible to certain diseases.

Genetic engineering has been a hot subject for many years. Research in genetic engineering has led to improvements in agricultural crop technology, and the manufacturing of synthetic human insulin through the use of modified bacteria.

Will advances in gene therapy and genetic engineering someday provide the keys to unlocking our vast lifespan? Possibly, but it is important to remember that the human body is a very complex organism. Many questions concerning genes and their effect on the human body still remain unanswered. Although research continues to make forward strides, it must be tempered by respect for what "Mother Nature" has already accomplished and the knowledge that the artificial manipulation of genes has the potential to backfire.

Neuroendocrine Theory

The Neuroendocrine Theory was first proposed in 1954 by the well-known Russian gerontologist Vladimir Dilman. Professor Dilman believed that the cause of aging could be traced directly to the loss of sensitivity that occurred in the hypothalamus, a walnut sized gland located in the brain. A great many hormones—needed to repair and regulate our body's functions—are regulated by the hypothalamus. The hypothalamus controls high-level chain reactions that instruct organs and glands like the pituitary, pineal, and thymus glands to release hormones to our body as needed.

The pituitary gland secretes HGH (human growth hormone) to regulate growth, TSH (thyroid-stimulating hormone) to regulate thyroid hormones, ACTH (adrenocorticotropic hormone) to regulate the adrenal glands, and FSH (follicle-stimulating hormone) and LH (luteinizing hormone) to regulate estrogen, testosterone, and progesterone.

The pineal gland, also located in the brain, secretes melatonin, which regulates sleep patterns. In the chest, just behind the breastbone, is the thymus gland, which stimulates certain infection-fighting cells to boost the immune system.

As we age, our hormone levels decline. This translates to the body's reduced ability to regulate and repair itself. Much like an old car that requires regular tune-ups and maintenance, the body depends upon the optimal hormone levels in order to function at its best. Without such care to the car, it runs the risk of breaking down very quickly. If done correctly, replacing the declining hormones helps to slow down or even reverse the aging process in our bodies.

Free Radicals and Oxidative Stress Theory

The Free Radical and Oxidative Stress Theory was developed by Dr. Denham Harman and introduced during the 1950s. Since then it has become widely regarded as one of the most popular and influential theories on the aging process, helping to spark strong public interest in the concepts of anti-aging, age-related diseases, and antioxidant supplementation. Today terms like "free radicals" and "antioxidants" are a part of our common vocabulary, but in order to go beyond the buzzwords and learn more about this concept we need to explore some of the lesser known functions of the body, beginning with electrons.

Electrons are required to produce electricity. The body also has an electrical system that utilizes electrons to perform its many vital functions, such as contraction of the heart and skeletal muscles, as well as to ensure that each one of the body's organs and tissues work properly.

A car burns gasoline in order to produce energy, creating toxic exhaust as a by-product. The body behaves in much the same way, burning sugar to produce energy in a process called oxidation. One of the main side effects of oxidation is the production of extra electrons, called free radicals, which are the body's own toxic exhaust. Unfortunately, extra free radicals circulating in the body attack and interfere with the functions of our cells. This free radical damage is called oxidative stress, which starts as soon as we are born. When we are young, the body has high levels of hormones to combat this oxidative stress and reduce the inflammation caused by the free radicals. As we grow older, our dropping hormone levels are not able to protect us from the damage of free radicals to our tissues, leading to inflammation, tissue destruction, and aging.

Environmental toxins can also pose a hazardous threat, acting either like free radicals in the body or by directly damaging our cells, or by a combination of both these negative effects. As we age, we are exposed to more toxins. Our environment, compared to the past, has many more chemicals that infiltrate into our water systems, consumer products, and the air. Many of these chemicals are not biodegradable, meaning that they will continue to persist in our environment for generations to come. The long-term impact these new toxins have on our planet and the human race has yet to be determined.

Substances that neutralize free radicals and prevent the harmful effects of oxidation are known as antioxidants. Eating fruits and vegetables supplies natural antioxidants to combat damage from free radicals. Other beneficial substances, called free radical scavengers, seek out free radicals and bind them before they attack body cells. Many vitamins and minerals have this function. Accordingly, if we can reduce the damage generated by free radicals and oxidative stress, we can slow down the aging process.

Other Theories

Mitochondrial Depletion

The energy producers for our body are tiny mitochondria that are found in each cell. When mitochondria quit working due to DNA damage, toxins, nutritional deficiency, or hormonal imbalance, we become very fatigued. Loss of mitochondrial energy production will lead to cell and tissue death.

Chronic Inflammation

Recent research has identified chronic inflammation as a common, underlying factor in several age-related diseases such as Alzheimer's disease, heart disease, diabetes and arthritis. Inflammation is our body's first line of defense against infection. When we are hurt or injured, immune cells quickly respond in order to prevent the spread of infection and repair damaged tissue. However, chronic inflammation, which can be caused by oxidative stress, chronic infection, accumulated toxins or hormonal imbalance, mistakenly signals our immune systems to continue this process, turning a healthy mechanism for healing into a continued assault upon otherwise healthy body structures. Left unchecked, this process can lead to a host of ill effects that help speed up the aging process.

Digestive Enzyme Deficiency

Digestive enzymes play a central role in our body's ability to break down and process the food we eat. Through the chemical reactions they create, our food is converted into the essential nutrients that our bodies require in order to build and repair cells, tissues, and organs. As we age, the number of digestive enzymes we are able to secrete declines, a process that eventually leads to inefficient digestion and absorption of nutrients. Without the ability to fully utilize vital nutrients, our body cannot function optimally, allowing the aging process to accelerate at a much faster rate.

Circulatory Deficiency

The circulatory system is our body's super-highway. This amazing infrastructure—composed of the heart, blood and blood vessels—connects all of the body's cells and is responsible for transporting nutrients, oxygen and water throughout the body.

A healthy, functioning circulatory system is critical to our body's ability to maintain optimum health. When the circulatory system's ability to deliver crucial nutrients is hampered, a number of problems can develop. Atherosclerosis for example, a hardening of the arteries, leads to poor circulation due to narrowing of the blood vessels. Reduced circulation to the capillaries in the eyes can lead to blindness, and reduced circulation to the brain can cause senility. Like an irrigation canal to crops, reduced circulation in our bodies leads to worn out and poorly performing organs.

Summary

Normal aging and pathological aging or premature aging are different. Normal aging is a process that occurs in every living organism. Our bodies are no exception to this rule, and normal age progression is recognized as a part of the cycle of life. However, pathological or premature aging is quite different. It is not a normal aging process and is brought on by diseases such as Alzheimer's, diabetes, heart disease and strokes, conditions that are largely preventable by improving the health and quality of our lifestyles.

The causes of premature aging are quite similar to the root causes of diseases. Many of the causative factors involved in the disease process lie in the choices we make everyday. Poor nutrition, obesity, lack of exercise, excessive tobacco and alcohol consumption and over-reliance on medications contribute to a large portion of this process. The power to change begins with us, and we can make the decision to take positive steps toward better health today, by making simple adjustments to our daily habits and lifestyle choices.

Making the commitment to achieve emotional balance and reduce the stress in our lives is critical as well. The time and effort we spend detoxifying our negative emotions and minimizing stressors at work and home will pay lasting dividends. These self-empowering choices will help form the foundation of optimum health.

As we progress further in the healing process—improving our nutrition, minimizing our exposure to toxins, detoxifying our bodies, reducing oxidative stress and balancing our hormones—we will largely prevent diseases, slow the aging process and dramatically enhance the quality of our lives.

Part II:

Hormone Balance

CHAPTER 3

Menopause and Bio-identical Hormone Replacement Therapy

Making the transition through menopause can be a turbulent and distressing time for women. The physical discomfort, emotional unrest, and lack of energy that accompany this midlife process can take a huge toll on women's vitality, usually when they need it the most.

Every day I see women in my office with similar stories. They have worked hard all of their lives either raising families, or as business professionals, or both. Now they have reached menopause and without warning their lives have suddenly started to deteriorate. Hot flashes keep them awake at night and the interrupted sleep leads to fatigue. They gain weight, even with more exercise and less food. Their moods become crabby and irritable. They are unable to concentrate and have poor memories due to foggy minds. They experience increasing vaginal dryness that makes intercourse painful, which many times is enough to kill any libido that remains. Their skin becomes dry and itchy, wrinkles creep up on their face, their breasts sag, and more fat begins to accumulate around their abdominal area. They look in the mirror and are horrified at what they have become.

Some choose to suffer through these symptoms in silence without getting any type of hormone replacement treatment due to fear of breast cancer. Some try over-the-counter remedies such as Estroven, black cohosh, or progesterone cream. Some are treated with birth control pills, antidepressants, or sleeping pills. Some receive conventional hormone treatment with Premarin® and/or progestin. Others try bio-identical hormone treatment with hormone creams, patches or gels.

The patients who come to see me often do so because the treatments they have tried have had little effect or bothersome side effects. They have heard from friends that the treatments I have applied have changed their lives. Thanks to treatment with bio-identical hormone implanted pellets their friends now sleep better without hot flashes or night sweats, their energy levels have soared, their moods are improved, and their libido is back. It is easier for them to lose weight and best of all they feel young again. Their sense of well-being has returned and they no longer feel trapped in a menopausal state.

Naturally these women come with all sorts of questions. If this is such a wonderful treatment, why haven't their doctors told them about it? Is it safe? Will it cause breast cancer? How are the hormone pellets implanted under the skin? How long do they last? What types of side effects occur? These are good questions, and their answers will help you better understand this effective treatment for any menopausal symptoms you may be experiencing. Let us start by examining the basic physiology of hormones. This information will assist you in understanding the variety of treatment options available so that you can make an informed decision when it comes to choosing the safest, most effective form of hormone replacement for your needs.

What Are Sex Hormones?

The Sex hormones consist of three types—estrogens, progesterone, and testosterone. Both men and women have all three hormones, but estrogen is predominant in women and testosterone is predominant in men.

Sources of Sex Hormones

1. **Ovaries:** The ovaries are the body's primary source of estrogen and progesterone before menopause. There are three forms of estrogen in the human body. They are estrone (E1), estradiol (E2), and estriol (E3). As you can see from the figure below, they show only a slight difference in their molecular structures. However, these subtle differences lead to quite important distinctions in the roles they perform.

Natural Estrogens

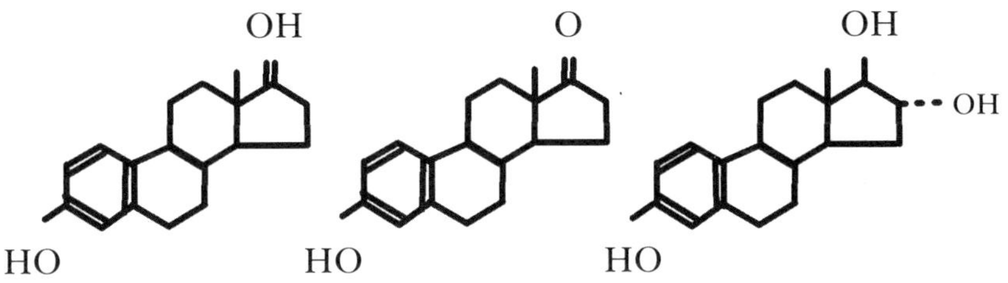

OH O OH
OH
HO HO HO

Estradiol (E2) Estrone (E1) Estriol (E3)

Figure 1. Natural estrogens.

Before menopause the ovaries mostly secrete estradiol, which accounts for the functions of estrogen we see in young women. Most of the positive effects of estrogen are due to estradiol. Estriol is produced in large amounts during pregnancy. It is a weak form of estrogen. Estrone and estradiol have to be metabolized into estriol before they can be excreted from the body. Our body needs estradiol to restore the normal physiology we had before menopause.

Ovaries secrete progesterone only after ovulation, which happens at mid-cycle. After menopause the ovaries discontinue production of estrogen and progesterone, but continue to produce testosterone.

2. **Adrenal glands:** The adrenal glands produce DHEA, a hormone precursor that can convert into testosterone. They also produce pregnenolone, which can convert into cortisol, DHEA, progesterone, testosterone and estrogen. Their contribution is critically important as they produce up to 30 percent of the sex hormone production in our younger years, and after menopause become the major source of sex hormone production.

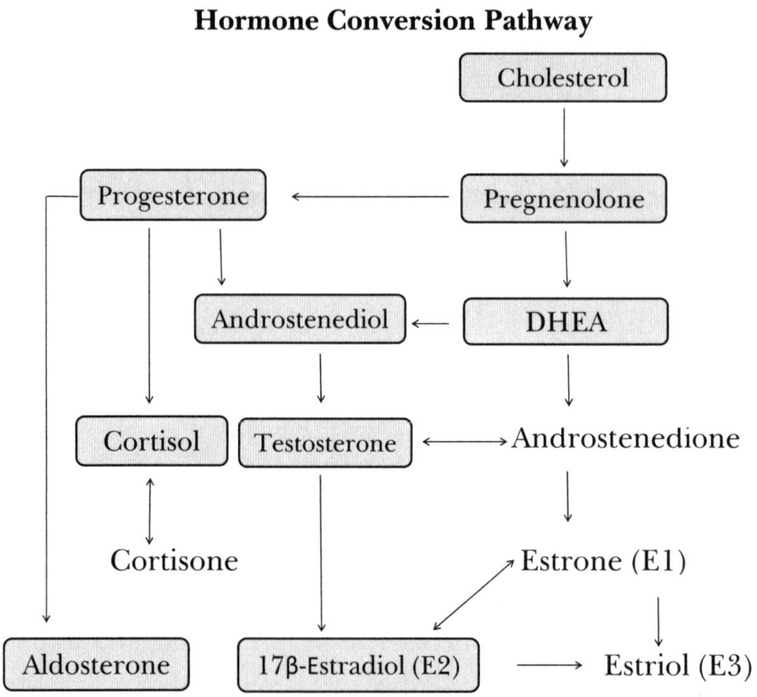

Hormone Conversion Pathway

Cholesterol

Progesterone ← Pregnenolone

Androstenediol ← DHEA

Cortisol

Testosterone ←→ Androstenedione

Cortisone

Estrone (E1)

Aldosterone

17β-Estradiol (E2) → Estriol (E3)

Figure 2. Hormone conversion pathways.

3. **Fat cells:** Fat cells, especially those found in the abdominal area, can produce hormones. They secrete estrone. There is a theory that women gain fat after menopause in order to compensate for the demand of estrogen in the body. Researchers have found that the ratio of estrone to estradiol changes after menopause. Whereas higher levels of estradiol are found in the body before menopause, that balance shifts to higher levels of estrone after menopause.

What Are the Functions of Sex Hormones?

Estrogen

1. **Reproductive organs:** The reproductive organs of the female body—the breasts, ovaries, vagina and uterus—all depend on the growth hormone estrogen. Without estrogen the body is negatively affected in numerous ways. For instance, breasts lose their volume and begin to sag. The lining of the uterus

becomes atrophic (withered) and there are no more menstrual periods. Estradiol maintains the health of the cells of the vagina and urinary bladder, which reduces vaginal dryness and urinary problems such as infections or incontinence.

2. **Cardiovascular system:** Estradiol is necessary for the health of the cardiovascular system. It dilates blood vessels, reducing blood pressure and limiting the formation of arteriosclerotic plaque on blood vessel walls. Loss of this estrogen is one of the reasons women tend to develop hypertension and cardiovascular disease after menopause.

   Insufficient estradiol also causes heart palpitations. Many women spend a lot of time and money having their hearts checked because of palpitations, only to discover that nothing is wrong and that the palpitations go away with adequate hormone replacement therapy.

3. **Central nervous system:** Estradiol increases the blood flow to the brain protecting nerve cells and brain function. It has a deep impact on our central nervous system. By increasing neurotransmitters such as acetylcholine and serotonin, estradiol helps with memory, relieves anxiety and depression, as well as promotes a normal sleep pattern. The sharp drop in estradiol makes it easy to see why many menopausal women complain of insomnia, anxiety, irritability, the inability to concentrate and lack of mental alertness.

4. **Skeletal system:** Estradiol is also vital to the skeletal system. It reduces bone loss and helps our body make new bones. Lack of estrogen and other sex hormones in the long-term leads to brittle bones, a condition we call osteopenia, and as it progresses becomes osteoporosis. Estradiol also improves the connective tissues in the joints, thereby reducing the likelihood of the onset of degenerative arthritis.

5. **Skin and hair:** Estradiol helps to promote smoothness and elasticity of the skin, improves skin dryness and prevents the loss of subcutaneous fat and collagen. Lack of it also leads to hair loss.

Progesterone

1. **Balances estrogen:** Progesterone helps to balance the effects of estrogen in the uterus and breast. Secreted by the ovaries after ovulation, it prevents overgrowth of the endometrium, the inner lining of the uterus. Menopausal women on HRT who still have a uterus need to take progesterone to prevent excessive buildup of the endometrium, which can lead to a heavy period and increase the possibility of getting endometrial cancer.

2. **Protects the nervous system:** Progesterone protects nerve cells and brain functions, and increases gamma-aminobutyric acid (GABA), a neurotransmitter that keeps us calmer and more relaxed. It also helps to restore normal sleep patterns.

3. **Natural diuretic:** Progesterone helps to prevent fluid retention by working as a natural diuretic.

4. **Optimizes estrogen receptors:** Lastly, progesterone helps estrogen receptors to function better.

Since nature designed progesterone to balance estrogen, much like the yin and yang, it is vital that levels of both hormones reach equilibrium to help maintain health. Estrogen dominance (excessive estrogen compared to progesterone), especially from environmental xenoestrogens, leads to fibrocystic breast disease, fibroid tumors, and even endometrial or breast cancer. When estrogen and progesterone are not balanced after ovulation, it leads to premenstrual tension, which includes such symptoms as heavy menstrual flow, fluid retention, moodiness, and migraine headaches.

Testosterone

Testosterone, considered by many to be a male sex hormone, is also important in women's health. Testosterone affects the body in many ways:

It increases muscle mass.
It boosts libido.
It assists in bone building and helps prevent osteoporosis.
It plays a very important role in protecting the cardiovascular system.
It helps with mood and works as an antidepressant.
It also helps keep the mind focused and sharp.
It promotes sensitivity to insulin and improves carbohydrate metabolism.

Testosterone's role in men's health has been well researched. Yet, the role of testosterone in women's health has long been neglected. This is tragic when in fact; testosterone plays the same roles in both men and women. Women, however, only have about 10 percent of the amount of testosterone as occurs in men, which is why women in general are neither as aggressive nor muscular as men.

The body's production of testosterone drops by about half between the ages of 30 and 50. Since the ovaries continue to produce testosterone after menopause, women do not experience the dramatic drop in testosterone that they do with estrogen and progesterone.

Bio-identical versus Synthetic Hormones

Both bio-identical hormones and synthetic hormones are produced by pharmaceutical companies and are FDA (Food and Drug Administration) approved. Bio-identical hormones have molecular structures that are exactly the same as the body's hormones. Synthetic hormones mimic the body's hormones, but are not an exact match. When using hormone replacement, it makes sense to use bio-identical hormones, since they have virtually the same chemical structures as those made by the human body. Examples of bio-identical estrogens that have been available to date are: Estrace®, Estradiol, Vivelle-Dot® patch, Climara® patch, bi-estrogen (bi-est) natural hormone cream or tri-estrogen (tri-est) natural hormone cream.

Typically, bio-identical hormones are derived from plant sources such as yams or soy. Unfortunately, humans do not have the enzymes in their bodies to convert these substances into bio-identical hormones, so adding soy or yams to your diet will not raise your hormone levels. Rather, these hormones must be synthesized in such a way so that they can be delivered safely in the body, such as with implanted pellets.

Hormones function by fitting into their own unique receptors that are on the membranes of the cells. Synthetic hormones that are not exactly identical to our own do not fit as well into the receptors and therefore may not be able to perform optimally. In addition, they can also produce side effects. Using them is comparable to opening a door with a copy of key that is not identical to the original key—it may not open the door, or may open a wrong door.

The synthetic hormones Premarin® and Provera® are the most commonly used forms of hormone replacement therapy and the most studied to date. Premarin® is a brand name that stands for "pregnant mare's urine" and is produced by Wyeth Pharmaceuticals and has been in use since its introduction in the 1950s. This hormone medication is manufactured by keeping a mare in a constant state of pregnancy and inserting a catheter into the horse's urinary bladder to collect her urine. It is from this urine that "conjugated equine estrogen" is extracted, which is approximately 75 percent estrone (E1) and 10 other forms of horse estrogens. The estrogen secreted by premenopausal women is primarily estradiol (E2), not estrone (E1). Replacing estrone instead of estradiol does not restore a woman's premenopausal physiology.

Provera® (or medroxyprogesterone) belongs to a class of drugs that are termed "progestins," which are synthetic progesterone. While it is supposed to perform the functions of progesterone, since it is not bio-identical, it can cause many negative side effects.

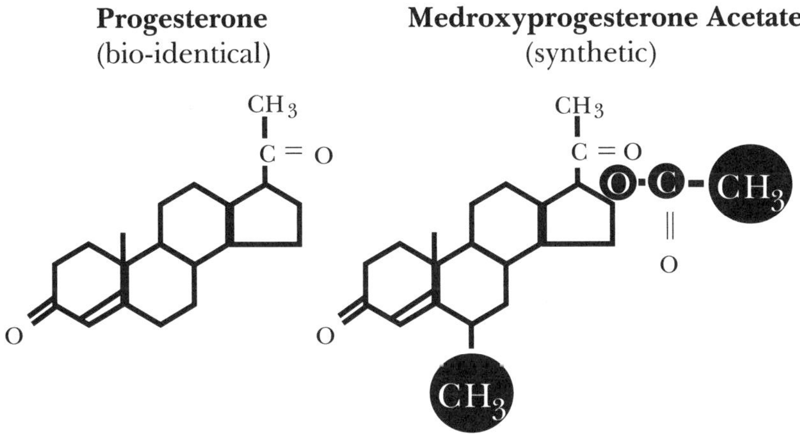

Figure 3. The molecular differences that create functional changes.

Synthetic progestins were originally developed to be more potent and longer-lasting than natural equivalents. They are also patentable by the pharmaceutical companies that make them. It is important not to confuse progestins with progesterone since their actions are so different.

Bio-identical hormone replacement is clearly superior to conventional synthetic hormone replacement because of its nearly perfect similarity to the hormones the body naturally produces. That is why it is called bio-identical.

Why Do We Need Hormone Replacement Therapy?

The most common reason women seek hormone replacement therapy (HRT) is the many miserable symptoms that typically accompany menopause. Women suffer from hot flashes, which can be socially embarrassing during the day and usually wake them up in the middle of the night. This leads to poor quality of sleep and fatigue. They gain weight due to the slowdown in metabolism associated with diminished hormone levels. Additionally many suffer from moodiness, depression, anxiety, poor memory, lack of concentration and mental fog. At the same time, women suffer from lack of libido and painful intercourse, but are often too embarrassed to complain of these symptoms to their doctors.

The second reason women need HRT is to help prevent, as well as treat, diseases that are related to aging. Studies have shown HRT improves blood sugar control in patients with diabetes, lowers blood pressure in patients with hypertension, delays the onset and decreases the risk of Alzheimer's disease, reduces age related eye diseases such as macular degeneration, reduces the risk of colorectal cancer, and prevents osteoporosis and fracture.[1,2,3,4,5,6,7,8] If you have a family history of diabetes, hypertension, dementia, macular degeneration, colorectal cancer or osteoporosis, utilizing hormone replacement therapy is an important step you can take to prevent these deadly diseases.

The third reason to consider HRT is its ability to slow down the aging process. Aging is significantly accelerated by hormone decline. By keeping hormones in the ranges we had during our 30s and 40s, we can maintain our vitality, youthful appearance and retard the aging process.

A century ago human life expectancy was 50 years; now it is about 80 years. It may even become 100 years in the not-so-distant future. Thirty or more years of low hormone levels may well lead to a miserably poor quality of life. Imagine lying in a nursing home bed, wearing a diaper, and being confused most of the time. It is not a pretty picture.

Hormone replacement therapy relieves the suffering that comes with menopause. Adequate hormone therapy gives people the assurance that they can enjoy life well into their golden years by preventing many of the diseases that accompany the aging process.

Breast Cancer and Hormone Replacement Therapy (HRT)

The most common reason women do not want HRT is due to the fear of breast cancer. Conventional thinking about hormones and breast cancer does not extend much beyond estrogen. As a matter of fact, there are many hormones that affect breast cancer in many different ways both positively and negatively. Those hormones include estrogens, progesterone, testosterone, DHEA, melatonin, oxytocin, insulin, T3 (thyroid hormone) and human growth hormone (HGH). It is important to pay attention to the levels of all these hormones when considering HRT.

Estrogen

- The Women's Health Initiative (WHI) study was designed to identify the potential benefits and risks of hormone replacement therapy (HRT). This study revealed that women who received estrogen only (Premarin®) did not have an increase in the occurrence of breast cancer. Only women who received Provera® in addition to Premarin® in the form of Prempro® had an increase in breast cancer risk.[7,9]

- A Swiss HRT study of 23,000 women, most of them using estradiol rather than conjugated equine estrogens (Premarin®), showed an actual decrease in the death rate from breast cancer.[10]

- Two studies out of MD Anderson demonstrated that estrogen use in women with a prior history of breast cancer showed a lower recurrence rate compared to the control group.[11,12]

- A review article analyzed 24 studies on women with a prior history of breast cancer published from 1986 to 2001. The recurrence rate of breast cancer and mortality rate were compared in women who received HRT versus women who did not receive HRT after breast cancer treatment. The meta-analysis (combining the data from all 24 studies and analyzing them together) showed that breast cancer survivors using HRT experienced a slightly reduced (8.2%) breast cancer recurrence rate, and an almost 4 times reduction in mortality rate.[13]

Although it is recognized that postmenopausal women with breast cancer tend to have higher blood levels of estrogen, what is not generally appreciated is that postmenopausal women have 10 to 50 times higher levels of estrogen in the breast than in the blood.[14,15] Fat cells around postmenopausal breast cancer have been found to have a high aromatase activity, which converts testosterone into estrogen, thereby generating it locally and increasing the rate of breast cancer cell growth. So exogenous estrogen does not cause cancer, but higher levels produced locally in the breast tissue, fuels the growth of existing cancer cells.

Our detoxification system plays an important role in cancer prevention. Premarin® blocks the important Phase II detoxification enzyme, glutathione S-transferase.[16] This blocking action of a critical detoxification step helps explain why Premarin® does not show the same breast protective effect that estradiol does. Studies have also shown that metabolites of equine estrogens cause oxidative damage to DNA, which also helps explain how long term use of Premarin® is linked to breast cancer.[17]

Progesterone

Progesterone appears to be an anti-breast cancer hormone. Several studies have been published that support the existence of this effect.

- A prospective epidemiological study done at Johns Hopkins Hospital demonstrated the protective role of natural progesterone against breast cancer. They followed 1,083 women who were evaluated and treated for infertility for 13 to 33 years. The results showed that the breast cancer rate was 5.4 times higher in women who had a lower progesterone level compared to those with a normal progesterone level.[18]

- Application of progesterone gel to the breast has been shown to reduce the growth activity of the breast glands.[19]

- Studies have demonstrated that in progesterone receptor positive breast cancer cells, progesterone regulates the gene expression and results in cancer cell death.[20,21,22]

It must be emphasized only bio-identical progesterone has those anti-cancer effects, not synthetic progestins such as medroxyprogesterone. Unfortunately, most medical literature does not distinguish between natural and synthetic progesterone and most physicians believe progesterone and progestins are the same thing, when in fact, the minimal change in the natural molecules that transform it into a progestin, changes the entire action and function of the molecule.

We also know estrogen helps with good health in the areas of mood, memory, blood pressure and the cardiovascular system. So why did the WHI study produces such discouraging results as increased cardiovascular complications, stroke and dementia? It is very likely that some of the complications were related to the use of medroxyprogesterone (a synthetic progestin), rather than bio-identical progesterone.

— Articles show that medroxyprogesterone increases the progression of coronary artery heart disease and causes insulin resistance and subsequent hyperglycemia.[23,24] Both of these outcomes are related to diabetes.

— In a study published in *The American Journal of Cardiology*, researchers studied two groups of postmenopausal women who had coronary heart disease. Both groups used estradiol (E2) for two weeks, then one group received intravaginal progesterone and the other group received oral progestin. Treadmill exercise tests were performed before hormone treatment as a baseline, 2 weeks after use of estradiol alone, and then at 10 days after adding progesterone or progestin. The study found that patients exercised on the treadmill longer without chest pain (myocardial ischemia) when they took two weeks of estradiol compared to their baselines. After adding bio-identical progesterone, the benefit of longer exercise time persisted, but with the use of synthetic progestin the benefit disappeared.[25]

Testosterone

Testosterone has been shown to have a direct anti-breast cancer effect. Consider the evidence below:

- A NIH (National Institutes of Health) study demonstrated that testosterone decreases the activities of breast cancer cells in monkeys.[26]

- In Italy, researchers demonstrated that testosterone inhibits breast cancer cells through it is own hormone receptor.[27]

In a clinical setting, this means that the addition of testosterone, along with progesterone, has the benefit of breast cancer protection. However, if someone has a very high aromatase enzyme in the breast, the situation may be different.

DHEA

Low DHEA levels have been associated with higher breast cancer risk in premenopausal women; on the other hand, however, high DHEA levels have also been associated with a higher incidence of breast cancer.[28] So for the time being, the best strategy is to keep DHEA levels within the normal range.

Melatonin

Melatonin is not just a sleep hormone; it also has anti-inflammation and anti-cancer effects. Night shift workers, such as nurses, tend to have lower melatonin levels and higher rates of breast cancer.[29] Using melatonin in a physiological dose should be considered in all women suffering from insomnia.

Many women are fearful about using HRT and choose instead to suffer silently with a poor quality of life and ongoing battles with age related diseases. Yet, balanced hormone replacement therapy does not increase the rate of breast cancer and may even help to reduce it.

Hormone Replacement Therapy—Routes of Delivery

Not all hormone replacement therapies are created equal. Although they all claim to treat menopausal symptoms, the way that they go about doing it can differ widely, not just in formulation (i.e., natural vs. synthetic), but also in the way they are applied and maintained. For the informed individual seeking relief from menopausal and mid-life hormonal deficiencies, the secret to success is finding a safe and effective method of hormone replacement.

Routes of Delivery Options

1. Oral.

When taking any medication orally, it is first absorbed in the GI (gastrointestinal) tract, after which 90 percent of the medicine goes directly to the liver. This is known as "first-pass metabolism."

Before menopause, our ovaries secrete hormones directly into the bloodstream through the capillaries. These hormones do not go to the liver first. Rather, they go directly to wherever they are needed in the body, undiluted and at full-strength. It is only after the body has used what it needs that any excess hormones are sent to the liver for excretion.

Estrogen taken orally reverses this normal route of hormone metabolism. The liver sequesters so much in its attempt of detoxifying the hormones; higher doses are required than our body actually needs in order to have a high enough concentration in the blood for the medication to do the job.

Additionally, estrogen taken orally increases the inflammation and clotting factors made in the liver. Studies have shown that bypassing the oral route with transdermal or implanted hormones does not negatively impact these cardiovascular risk factors.[30,31] These consequences reveal why taking estrogen orally is not the best way to receive hormone replacement.

2. Transdermal.

Transdermal methods of delivery involve direct application to the skin. This is usually accomplished by using hormone creams, gels, or patches. Currently two bio-identical estrogen (E2) patches (Vivelle-Dot® and Climara®) have been made available. A transdermal form of the bio-identical progesterone patch has not yet been developed. Testosterone patches are available for men, but not for women. One drawback of patches is that they have adhesives that can cause skin irritation. Creams or gels have to be applied at least once a day, and they can be messy. Compliance is a concern, since people tend to forget to apply the cream, particularly if their memories are not very good. Absorption is another issue, which is affected by each individual's skin condition and the mixing substance used to manufacture the cream or gel. Creams can be useful for women if their skin absorption is adequate and they remember to consistently apply the cream.

3. Sublingual.

Sublingual lozenges or troches under the tongue deliver hormones directly through the tissues in the mouth. The sublingual route of delivery causes a surge of hormones that diminishes within eight to twelve hours. Many people cannot handle this surge of hormones.

Progesterone is the only hormone I give my patients in the sublingual form, since it helps people sleep at night and does not cause drowsiness during the day.

4. Suppositories.

Intravaginal or rectal suppositories can also be used to deliver hormones, but due to the discomfort involved many women dislike this route.

5. Injections.

Intramuscular injections cause a surge of hormones that diminishes quickly, and require weekly or monthly injections. A significant drawback with this method of delivery is that bio-identical hormones are not available for injections.

6. Subcutaneous (beneath the skin) Pellet Implants.

This is the most physiologically appropriate form of hormone replacement. It is as if your own ovaries are functioning again. The many benefits of this route of hormone replacement are discussed in detail in Chapter 4.

The following chart, figure 4, illustrates the absorbability of different hormone delivery routes. As you can see pellet implants have the greatest absorption over long-term

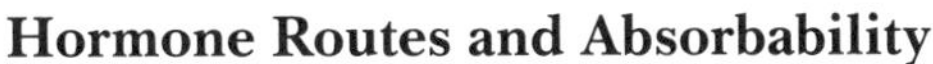

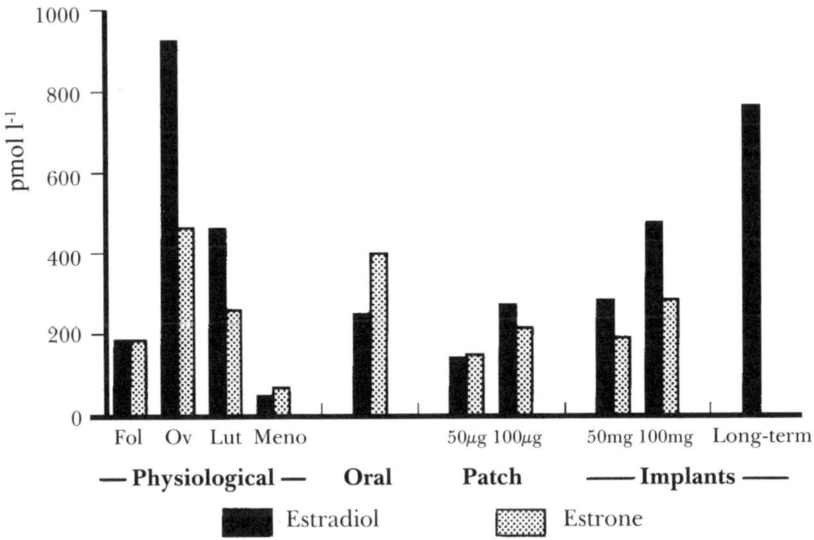

Fol = Follicular
Ov = Ovulatory
Lut = Luteal
Memo = Menopausal

Mean hormone concentrations achieved with different routes of estrogen delivery. (Englund, et al., 1977; Thom, et al., 1981; Powers, et al., 1985; Garnett, et al., 1990; Stanczyck, 1991).

Source: Studd JW and Smith RN. Oestradiol and testosterone implants. *Baillières Clin Endocrinol Metab.* 1993;7(1):203-223. Reprinted with permission.

Figure 4. Mean hormone concentrations.

Rules of Hormone Replacement

The use of hormone replacement therapy requires paying attention to important details. Here are the guidelines:

1. If you need hormone replacement, use bio-identical hormones that are delivered through physiological routes, such as through the skin or implanted beneath the skin.

2. Remember that all of the body's hormones are interrelated. It is important to balance all hormones, including the sex, adrenal, and thyroid hormones.

3. Hormone levels must be monitored periodically in order to make sure that they are balanced and in the appropriate normal ranges.

There have been many studies published on hormone replacement therapy, The Women's Health Initiative Study being one of the most recent. Even though it produced negative results for the reasons we discussed above, many studies conducted in the past have demonstrated the ability of HRT to reduce heart disease and dementia. There are currently many ongoing studies of HRT, and when the cloud of dust from all the research finally settles in the next 20 to 30 years, I believe that the positive results we are seeing today will continue to be validated.

Women who use the right type of hormone replacement will experience an improved quality of life into their golden years by reducing heart disease, strokes, dementia, and osteoporosis. This is in addition to the benefits of reducing hot flashes, improving sleep, mood, memory, libido, and energy!

CHAPTER 4

Subcutaneous Bio-identical Hormone Pellet Implants

The Ultimate Hormone Replacement Therapy

The first documented instance of an implant for hormone replacement occurred in 1938 at Guy's Hospital in London. It was developed at that time for women who had undergone a radical hysterectomy (removal of uterus) and bilateral oophorectomy (removal of both ovaries). In spite of many apparent advantages over other delivery routes, such as oral medications or gels or patches, hormone pellets are only used by a few trained physicians in English-speaking countries such as the United Kingdom, Australia, South Africa and the United States. Physicians are trained to use hormone replacement therapy in the United States relying on hormone pills and patches manufactured and promoted by pharmaceutical companies. Many doctors are biased against bio-identical hormones and most doctors have not even heard about pellet therapy, but assume that they are just as bad as synthetic hormones, which does not appear to be true.

Dr. Gino Tutera, a board certified ob-gyn and founder of the SottoPelle® Society, has been implanting pellets as a bio-equivalent hormone replacement therapy for women over the last 15 years with great success. He has trained more than 100 physicians in the U.S. to perform this very simple, yet effective treatment. The SottoPelle® Society was formed in 2004 and I am one of the original members. Other physicians in the U.S. implant pellets too, but the dosages and methods vary somewhat.

Advantages of Pellet Therapy Demonstrated in Studies

Dr. John Studd in England published many papers on pellet implants and argued that the hormone profiles achieved and the efficacy of implant therapy should be used as a first-line therapy in patients with severe menopausal symptoms.[32,33] His studies, as well as others showed:

1. There was no evidence linking pellet therapy to an increased incidence of breast cancer.[34]

2. Orally administered estrogen is associated with altered coagulation factors and lipid panels while subcutaneously implanted pellets show no adverse effect on blood pressure, lipids, coagulation factors, and insulin and glucose metabolism.[35,36,37] As discussed in the previous chapter, this is because the subcutaneous implantation of hormone pellets bypasses the liver and avoids the induction of liver factors that can negatively impact the cardiovascular system.

3. Pellet therapy restores the 2:1 ratio of E2 to E1, which is the physiological balance of younger age women, and effectively improves bone density when compared to other methods of hormone replacement. Studd et al. demonstrated a four-fold increase (8.3%) in bone density in patients who received pellets compared to oral estrogen (2.8%) in postmenopausal women after 1 year of treatment.[38]

4. Pellet therapy promotes a more stable blood level compared to pills and patches. Oral estrogen has a roller coaster effect, while the patch is more stable but still goes up and down. Pellets are the only delivery method that provides stable E2 blood levels.

Blood Level Comparisons of Pellet Implants, Patch, and Oral

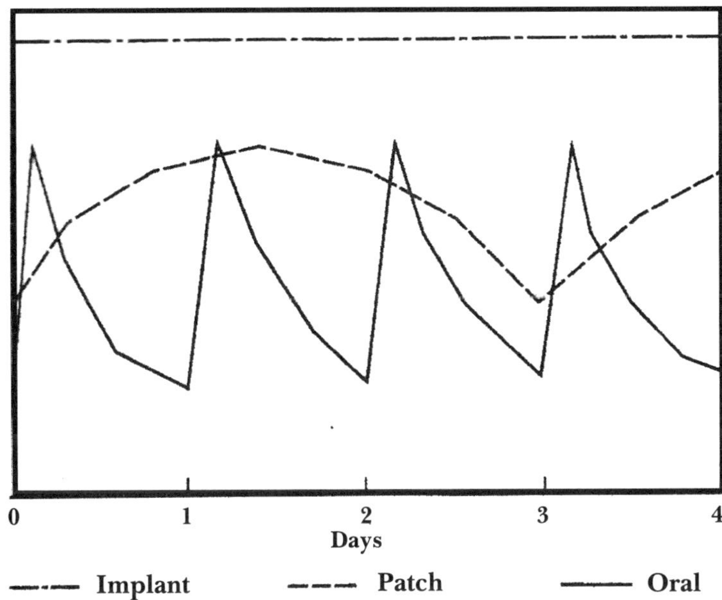

Figure 5. Short-term variation in estradiol concentrations with pellet implant, patch, and oral therapy.

Source: Studd JW and Smith RN. Oestradiol and testosterone implants. *Baillières Clin Endocrinol Metab.* 1993;7(1):203-223. Reprinted with permission.

5. Montgomery et al. demonstrated that estradiol implants were significantly more effective than placebo in relieving depression and anxiety in postmenopausal women.[39]

6. Testosterone implants help to improve libido and weight loss by building muscles. Other types of HRT usually do not use testosterone. Transdermal testosterone cream does not achieve the same results as implanted pellets.

7. Pellet therapy is hassle free—there are no creams to rub on every day or patches to replace once or twice a week.

Implant Procedure

Implanting pellets is an easy, quick and safe office procedure that is carried out under local anesthesia, so there is minimal to no pain involved. The skin is cleaned with an antiseptic and then numbed. A tiny incision (3 mm) is made and the pellets are inserted through a trochar (tool used to inject pellet) just under the skin, into the subcutaneous fat of either the lower abdominal wall or the outer quarter of the buttock. Afterward the incision is covered with a sterile strip. A stitch may be required only if there is excessive bleeding.

Biological Action of Implants

After implantation, there is a rapid rise of estradiol and a decline of follicular stimulating hormone (FSH), which is a hormone secreted by the pituitary gland to regulate estrogen. A high level of FSH means the body wants to stimulate the ovaries to produce more estrogen. A lower FSH level means the body feels that there is enough estrogen, so the ovaries do not need to be stimulated to make more.

The figures below show the decline in FSH and rise in E1 and E2 after a 50 mg pellet implantation, which is then followed by their respective gradual rise and fall.

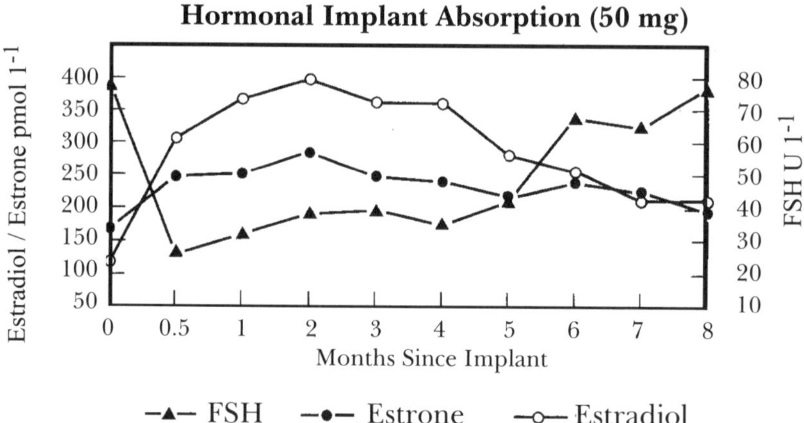

Figure 6. FSH, estrone and estradiol concentrations with 50 mg estradiol implant.

Source: Studd JW and Smith RN. Oestradiol and testosterone implants. *Baillières Clin Endocrinol Metab.* 1993;7(1):203-223. Reprinted with permission.

Frequently Asked Questions

1. How soon will I see the effects of pellet therapy? How long do the pellets last and how will I know when the pellets begin to run out?

My patients usually see effects within one week, some even in 1 to 2 days. The amount of time pellets last can vary with the individual, but it is usually between 4 to 6 months. While the original symptoms might not return together all at once, they will gradually reappear one by one, alerting patients to the fact that it is time for an implant again.

2. How does the body know to take the proper amount of hormones it needs?

Since a hormone pellet is surrounded by blood vessels under the skin, its rate of hormone release is regulated by the heart rate and cardiac output (the amount of blood pumped out of the heart with a single contraction). If you compare the body to a child licking a lollipop—the faster the heart rate—the more hormone is released—just like when a child licks a lollipop rapidly. The slower the heart rate the less hormone is released. As long as the heart is beating and there is a fragment of a pellet remaining, the hormone will be released to the body. Therefore, more hormone is released when the heart rate rises with either physical or emotional stress. When the physical (exercise, strenuous work) or emotional stress is no longer present the amount of hormone that is released from the pellet will decrease and return to the steady continuous flow provided by a normal heart rate. The amount of hormone released is also dependent upon both the dosage as well as the hormone concentration difference between the pellet and blood vessel. A higher dosage (a larger size pellet) provides a greater contact surface that releases more hormone to the blood stream. A hormonally depleted body will also pull more hormone from the pellet since the concentration in the blood stream will be lower than the tissue surrounding the pellet.

With this method of hormonal delivery, the tissue hormone levels are stable 24 hours a day, seven days a week. Because the estrogen levels do not go too high or fluctuate, pellet therapy does not stimulate the breasts at the same level as synthetic hormones.

If a person is stressed and the body requires the support of more hormones, the pellets will be used more quickly. It is similar to having a full tank of gas in the car. If you drive a lot, the tank will empty out sooner. This is the only form of hormone therapy that can deliver more as needed.

3. What is in the pellets?

Pellets are made of bio-identical estradiol or testosterone. They are made in different dosages by compounding pharmacies; fused into the size of a grain of rice, sterilized, and stored in individual small glass containers. Progesterone should not be implanted because a woman's natural menstrual cycle only provides progesterone 50 percent of the time, not the 100 percent of the time that an implanted pellet would supply. Also, progesterone pellets would secrete continuously and be more likely to cause irregular bleeding.

4. Is it FDA approved?

A testosterone pellet called Testopel has recently been approved by the FDA. Bio-identical estradiol is approved by the FDA and currently made by compounding pharmacists who operate at all times with federal and state mandated guidelines.

5. Will my period return when I am on pellet therapy?

If your estrogen returns to levels you had at a younger age, and you use progesterone for only 2 weeks out of the month, you will have a period. It can actually be a good idea to have a period, as it helps to clean up the uterine linings. However, if you do not want to have your period back, take progesterone continuously—this suppresses the growth of the uterus lining and will prevent the occurrence of a period.

Indications for Pellet Therapy

Let us take a look now at some of the primary conditions and their symptoms that indicate a person's need for hormone replacement. Individual patient stories will also help to illustrate the effectiveness of pellet therapy in treating these conditions.

1. Menopause

The most common reason that people seek hormone replacement therapy is due to menopausal symptoms. These include:

Hot flashes and/or night sweats
Insomnia or poor quality of sleep
Fatigue
Moodiness, depression, and/or anxiety
Memory loss/forgetfulness
Difficulty concentrating
Lack of motivation
Heart palpitations
Hair loss
Vaginal dryness, painful intercourse, low libido
Urinary incontinence or infection
Aching joints and muscles
Bone loss/osteoporosis

All of these symptoms due to low hormone levels are relieved when implanted pellets deliver adequate hormone replacement.

2. Perimenopause

Laurie's story:

My name is Laurie, age 50, and a few years ago I became perimenopausal, which started with hot flashes that would wake me up at 3:30 or so every morning. I also noticed that I had no tolerance or patience for things that had not previously bothered me. Headaches and joint pains also started to occur. Since my older sister had already been going through menopause, I was aware that my symptoms meant I was in its early stages.

I am proactive about my health, including being very diligent about nutrition and exercising regularly. I was aware that weight gain usually comes with menopause. While that had not happened to me yet, I was concerned about it. So, I began reading books about menopause and found out about a hormone saliva test to determine if you are menopausal. My efforts to find someone to administer this test led me to Karen Sun, M.D. Sure enough, the test showed that I was indeed perimenopausal.

Other symptoms that had set in included less confidence and a lack of mental clarity. Until I became perimenopausal, I had been a very confident person, but suddenly I doubted myself on things that, before, I knew were a given. Things just no longer were making sense in my life. It is like in those commercials where the bird flies into the window. That is kind of how it feels being perimenopausal.

Dr. Sun and I decided to go with the pellets to alleviate my symptoms. After I had the pellets, I suddenly felt better. My frame of mind improved. I had more strength when I worked out at the gym, and the hormones balanced things out.

They have helped me get through the hills and valleys of life a lot more easily. It was as though one day someone lifted the shade that had covered your life. When you get your hormones right, everything becomes crystal clear, and I wondered why I had struggled with all that stuff before.

A female colleague talked about being perimenopausal, how there is nothing you can do about it, and that there is nothing you can take to feel better. I told her that is not true and talked with her about what Dr. Sun had done for me. We do not have to be miserable; we do not have to go through hot flashes, insomnia, or weight gain if we have pellets. I try to tell as many people about this as possible.

I recently had my skin evaluated for a special facial treatment, and the lady told me that I do not look anywhere near 50. She said, "Whatever you are doing, keep doing it." I think the hormones preserve us all the way around. I feel lucky that my research took me in the direction of Dr. Sun.

I want to be happy; I don't want to be miserable. I feel very blessed that I have been able to find Dr. Sun and experience this relief from menopausal symptoms. She has made my life so much better. She has put her heart and soul into helping her patients get their hormones balanced. I know she has changed the lives of many. I know for a fact that she has improved my quality of life.

When a woman is perimenopausal, or at the early stage of entering menopause, she will still have a menstrual period, but it will be very irregular. Hot flashes may or may not occur. The most bothersome symptoms are moodiness, especially immediately prior to the menstrual period; migraine headaches; and sleep disturbance. These symptoms are due to the fluctuation of hormone levels, especially when a woman is stressed and her body is not able to produce higher levels of hormones to meet the increased need.

I find that pellet implants with testosterone alone are very helpful in this situation, because testosterone stabilizes the estrogen levels by converting to estrogen at the cellular level. Testosterone is also very effective in relieving moodiness, low libido and fatigue symptoms, which happen quite often at this stage. In many women the same symptoms are treated with birth control pills, but the results achieved through implanted pellets are much more effective. If there is heavy bleeding or breast tenderness present, I will sometimes add progesterone cream or lozenges to address these symptoms.

3. Menstrual Migraines

Erica's story:

My name is Erica, and I started getting very severe migraines during my second pregnancy, which happened seven years ago. The headaches worsened progressively thereafter and typically occurred around my menstrual cycle. My doctor and the specialists to whom I had been referred put me on a lot of different medications, including injections and antidepressants. Nonetheless, I was still having migraine headaches that were so terrible they made me vomit. I even had to go to the hospital a couple of times. These headaches put me out of commission. They would last for days, and I was completely not functioning in life. I thought I was going to have to quit work, and I could not even take care of my children. Then I read a book called "The Hormone Solution," which is when I first heard about bio-identical hormones. At the time I lived in Connecticut and flew to California to see Dr. Sun. I was in very bad shape, but within a few days of having the pellets my migraines abated and I have not had a terrible migraine since. I have been able to go off of all the medications, including the antidepressants. The pellets have been the total miracle cure for me. I have been on the pellets for two years now and I have my life back. To be able to play with my kids again and function in life is really awesome.

Migraines are a common disorder affecting about 20 percent of all women. The fact that migraines usually start after puberty and 60 percent of these headaches are related to the menstrual period suggests that this is a hormone issue. I also find that testosterone implants are helpful for this condition, as it stabilizes the hormone levels. I have quite a few patients suffering from menstrual migraines who have tried other treatments without effect. Testosterone pellet implantation often helps them tremendously, as well as very small doses of estradiol in pellet form.

4. Osteoporosis

Amelia's story:

I am Amelia, 63, with a slender build and of Scandinavian descent. All of these factors are typical risks for osteoporosis. I went for my first bone density exam about 12 years ago. I was told at that time that I have thinning bones. So, I was put on various medications for this condition. Each year as I would have a bone density scan and would find out that my condition sometimes was better, or worse, depending on the type of medication I had been given. Then came the scare about taking estrogen, so I went off of it and used a hormone replacement therapy in the form of a cream. I also wanted to go off of the bone density medication after a CT scan showed that I had a lot of liver cysts.

This was when I went to Dr. Sun, who introduced me to the possibility of pellets. She is in favor of using the physiological route of delivery of bio-identical hormones by subcutaneous implantation instead of the oral delivery through the stomach and liver. I decided to try the pellets for a year to see what would happen. I received estrogen and testosterone pellets and sublingual progesterone. After a year, my bone density exam showed an increase of bone density in my hip and spine. This increase had to be as a result of the pellets, as was the only thing I was doing differently. Other bone meds will keep down deterioration of bone, but do not build new bone. Now I have had between 1.4% and 2.1% increases in bone density in various areas. What is more, my liver function has tested as normal. This is very encouraging.

Both estrogen and testosterone improve bone density. Pellet implant therapy supplies the body with a steady amount of hormones so it is more effective than other routes of hormone therapy in treating osteoporosis.

5. Depression and Anxiety

Vicki's story:

I am Vicki, 67, and I have been very healthy and active all my life, working out and playing tennis until age 50. I was running six miles a day. Then, menopause struck. My worst symptom was anxiety. I was married at the time to a physician who did not believe in hormone replacement therapy. He said it was unnatural and that I should just tough it out. Being the good wife, that is what I did. I have not been the type to be anxious and stay at home, but I became that way. I was afraid and very unsure of myself. Then, my husband died when I was 53. I became so anxious that it came to the point I could not function. It was a terrible time in my life. I sold my husband's medical practice to another physician, who told me to get on hormones. He started giving me synthetic estrogen injections. That worked all right for a few years until the controversy over hormones occurred. Even that doctor said then that I should get off the hormones. I finally stopped them and then I really started to feel bad. I had no libido; I became super anxious; I had no energy at all. I just dragged through the day. This went on for a full year until I found out about bio-identical hormone replacement therapy.

After I went on the pellets, I started to feel so much better—I became a different person. I had no more anxiety and I was stronger. I went back to being the way I was before menopause. The pellets have been tremendous. I am so rejuvenated and I have absolutely no side effects. I am back to playing golf, swimming, and walking at least four miles a day. All of my anxiety and other symptoms were a result of the lack of hormones. Once we got that under control, I became fine. This is wonderful. I feel healthy and good. I will continue to do this until I die.

The role of hormones in depression is well documented in patients with postpartum (after childbirth) depression and premenstrual syndrome. Pellet implants improve mood, especially depression and anxiety. In my clinical experience I have seen many patients who have been treated with antidepressants or tranquilizers before they have come to me. After pellet implantation, I have often been able to help them reduce or discontinue antidepressants and tranquilizers successfully.

6. Testosterone Deficiency and Sexual Dysfunction

Carey's story:

My name is Carey, 47, and for a couple of years before I found the pellets, I was absolutely uninterested in sex. Period. End of story. Any lovemaking I did with my husband was from a sense of duty. Now, with my hormones at a normal, healthy level, I have more of a sex drive. I no longer have to accept that losing interest in my sexuality is unavoidable and a part of growing older. I like feeling attractive and sensual again. It is great to have regained this special connection with my husband. I also like the mental clarity and getting up in the morning feeling rested. I like waking up with energy. Those are the benefits I feel from the pellets more than anything else.

Most women are embarrassed to admit how low libido bothers them. After pellet therapy, many women have told me that they have experienced such dramatic improvements in their sex lives that their husbands have talked about sending me flowers. Their husbands, in fact, are usually the ones who remind them they are due for pellets. Women, who once had no interest in dating, experience such a boost in their libido and self-confidence that they completely reinvigorated their social lives; in many cases they start dating and even get married after receiving pellet treatment.

Female androgen insufficiency syndrome (FAIS) widely exists but is rarely talked about. So far, it is a clinical diagnosis made from signs and symptoms. The clinical symptoms of FAIS include decreased libido and sexual pleasure, a diminished sense of well-being, depressed mood or lack of motivation, and persistent fatigue. Physical signs include bone loss, decreased muscle mass and reduced strength, which leads to more fat in the body.

The normal level for testosterone in women has not been well established. Premenopausal women produce 0.1 to 0.2 mg of testosterone daily and to maintain the normal function of the human body women must receive the equivalent amount of testosterone when receiving hormone therapy. Most labs use a normal value of 20 to 80 ng/dl, which is outdated. In a paper published out of Princeton University Medical School, a number of the world's experts on testosterone therapy for women found that all the assays used most frequently by the laboratories could not measure levels of testosterone below 300 ng/dl accurately.[40]

Additionally, hormone levels vary in different age groups, and no normal values for different age groups have been established. Furthermore, most testosterone is bound up with hormone-binding protein, and only the unbound component (free testosterone) is active. Testosterone testing is designed for men who have ten times more testosterone than women. So, this test becomes inaccurate when the free testosterone is measured at women's much lower levels. Another factor not often accounted for is the possibility of testosterone resistance, like insulin resistance, can affect the interpretation of test results. One may show sufficient hormone levels in a blood test but still have the symptoms of deficiency.

I find the most common cause of FAIS is adrenal fatigue. Remember, the adrenal glands secrete DHEA, which is the precursor to testosterone. Most women are so stressed in their daily lives that almost all of them suffer from adrenal fatigue, just with varying degrees of severity. Another reason for FAIS is surgical oophorectomy (removal of an ovary or both ovaries) or incidental injury to blood circulation in the ovaries due to other surgeries, such as hysterectomy or tubal ligation. Birth control pills by suppressing ovulation and reducing FSH (follicular stimulation hormone) result in reduced production of testosterone from the ovaries.

7. Adrenal Fatigue

Sarah's story:

I am Sarah, 74, a retired college professor. I was experiencing with increasing exhaustion, and when I read up on the adrenals I thought they could be a factor in my being so tired. Then I had three serious operations on my knees and neck over a two-and-a-half year period. I became so tired, had no energy, was depressed, and cried constantly. Everything was a monumental effort, and I am a high-energy person. When I walked into Dr. Sun's office a year ago, I was wiped out. My head was literally crouched over the steering wheel of my car. She could see that I was hanging by a thread. She gave me a small pellet insertion and we went from there. Little by little, she has brought me back to health. The pellets are a miracle and I could not live without them. I have been on them for a year now and never want to be without them again. We are working on building up my adrenals with the combination of pellets and supplemental medications, such as hydrocortisone and adrenal herbs. I do feel more energy and have more zest for life. This has been an incredible transformation, as I am now taking water aerobics classes and working in my garden again.

The reduced functioning of the adrenal glands is a modern disease due primarily to chronic stress and longer lifetimes. In Chapter 7 we will be talking about this epidemic in detail. I find that pellet therapy with testosterone is very helpful in relieving the symptoms of fatigue. Testosterone is one of the major sources of estrogen for women after menopause, since testosterone can convert into estrogen in the tissue. When women have their ovaries removed, they have a more difficult time coping with menopausal symptoms because after menopause the body depends on the ovarian production of testosterone. The same holds true for women who have adrenal fatigue, because decreased production of DHEA by the adrenal glands also results in low levels of testosterone.

8. Cystitis and Urinary Tract Infection

Andrea's story:

I am Andrea, aged 59, and I have had interstitial cystitis (IC), or painful bladder syndrome, for 25 years. This disease causes the pain and symptoms of a urinary tract infection, but it is not caused by bacteria. A million people in the U.S. have this disease, and 80 to 90 percent are female. Urologists have been searching for the answers of what causes IC. It is something wrong with the lining of the bladder. It certainly is life altering. Many people cannot work or leave their homes because of this disease. In many cases, it leads to suicide. It is just dreadful. I am lucky that my symptoms are moderate to severe and I have a high tolerance for pain, but this disease has been the bane of my existence. It comes on periodically. It hurts to urinate with IC; it is like being allergic to your own urine, and you have to go to the bathroom constantly. When I was diagnosed 25 years ago, the only treatment was a bladder wash that instills DMSO (dimethyl sulfoxide). It can bring relief, and I have had DMSO once every 6 weeks to 2 months. Then a new drug called Elmiron came out. Although it helps with IC symptoms, It can make you lose your hair. I like my hair, so I did not continue with this drug. For 15 years I have been on Elavil, an antidepressant that has the amazing benefit of blocking pain. I have kept the symptoms of IC reasonably under control with these three treatments. I also had a hysterectomy around the same time I was diagnosed with IC and one ovary was removed 2 years later. At first I was on Estrace® for hormone replacement therapy and then switched to another form of estradiol after a couple of years.

None of these hormone therapies made any difference at all with the IC symptoms. It never occurred to me to connect hormones with this disease. But when I started on the implanted bio-identical hormone pellet therapy with Dr. Sun a few years ago, all of my IC symptoms were suddenly reduced by about 70 percent. It was absolutely unbelievable. After the pellets were implanted, I went 6 months without DMSO bladder irrigation. Then I went 10 months without it. Naturally, I said something to my urologist about this link. He said he was not surprised because hormone therapy helps support the bladder. I cannot tell you the difference the pellet therapy has made in my life. I love the pellets for all the other obvious reasons. Everything is better with the pellets, but I would use them if for no other reason than they have changed the nature of this disease that I have had. My urologist gives women hormone creams, but that does not do it like the pellets. I tried them. There is something very different about the pellets that make them so much more effective. In addition, they make me feel more youthful.

Having provided pellet therapy to over 1,000 patients now, coupled with Dr. Tutera treating over 10,000 patients, we have both witnessed an amazing number of success stories. Andrea, with interstitial cystitis, is just one example. Some of my patients have tried multiple antidepressants without relief, only to find that pellet therapy is the only thing that alleviates their depression. Women suffering from fibromyalgia improve greatly with pellet therapy. Other women burdened by adrenal fatigue recovered after their sleeping patterns improved due to pellet therapy. The list of benefits goes on and on.

Best Candidates for Pellet Therapy

The following categories describe those groups of women who are generally best suited to benefit from pellet therapy.

1. **Women who have adrenal fatigue and become surgically menopausal with removal of both ovaries and the uterus.**

Elizabeth's story:

My journey began when I entered perimenopause at the age of 40. I now know that I was entering it early as my job was very demanding and I was in a stage of adrenal fatigue, as well as only had one functioning ovary. My primary symptom was very heaving bleeding with many clots being passed. Even though I had been in the medical profession my whole life, I did not understand my body well enough to know that it was progesterone that was lacking and natural progesterone would have probably corrected the problem. Instead I believed my doctor that estrogen would help and took the oral estradiol he prescribed. Over a course of 3 years the bleeding never improved and he told me that a hysterectomy was my only answer. I sought out a female gynecologist for a second opinion, and did not realize that doctors are trained with the same medical school training, as she agreed a hysterectomy was the only answer and told me "I would feel so better than ever afterwards." I trusted both of these opinions, especially since they agreed with each other, and at the age of

43 agreed to a hysterectomy. When I woke up with an estrogen pill being shoved down my throat, I found out the doctor also took my ovaries even though he had never once discussed this with me. When I asked why he took them, he told me, "Well you are over 40 and you don't want cancer in your future, do you?" I realized I could not put my ovaries back so I went home determined to feel so much better than ever afterwards.

Over the weeks and month that followed, however, I did not. I fell into a deep suicidal depression, my blood pressure was out of control even though it had been low normal my entire life, I had no energy and even quit going to work as all I could do was drag my body around all day, and sexually had lost all feeling and ability to respond. When I told my doctor about all these symptoms he told me it was all in my head and wanted to refer me to a psychiatrist. When I said, "No! This is chemical change!" he referred me to an endocrinologist who just changed my brand of oral estrogen and added progesterone cream.

After a year and a half, I finally found a doctor who understood the symptoms caused by loss of the ovaries. She explained that I was not absorbing the oral estrogen and she felt about 20 percent of women do not. She also helped me understand I must have been a high testosterone maker and was missing the testosterone as much if not more than the estrogen. As a result, she started me on combination estradiol and testosterone shots. These would make me feel like my old self for only about a day, so I was getting shots once a week. We tried estradiol and testosterone creams. These did not help me feel any better. She also explained that some women do not absorb creams, so I was one of those also. Then we tried the estradiol patches. I never felt good on them and was swimming everyday and I found they just floated off into the pool. After a year and a of working with her and still not feeling good every day, she said there was a company that was attempting to get FDA approval for hormone pellet implants. She explained they were compact pure hormone pellets that would be implanted under the skin. I was ready to try anything at this time, as I had not felt good the entire 3 years since my surgery. Even though I did not feel their effect for 2 weeks, when I finally started in feeling their effect I was elated, as it was the first time since surgery that I felt anywhere near close to my old self. That was in 1988 and I have been on them, almost consistently, since then.

There was a 2-year period of time when the company that made the pellets went bankrupt and I could not obtain them anymore. I tried several other manufacturers of the pellets, but was not absorbing them. At the time, I went back to the shots, the creams, and the patches and fell into all the same horrific symptoms I had felt after surgery. I was hot flashing and crying on a daily basis. Again I had no energy and no ability to respond sexually. At this time I also developed the excruciatingly painful symptoms of fibromyalgia as well as had osteoarthritis in my hands, which was so bad I could not hold hands with my husband and my joints had taken on the gnarled misshapen appearance of arthritic joints. I finally called my family practitioner and said, "You have got to find pellets for me. They are the only things that work for me." She found the pellets and within 2 weeks after implanting them the hot flashes, crying, and my fibromyalgia disappeared totally and completely. I was thrilled to feel good again and to understand that the fibromyalgia had been connected to just low estradiol and testosterone. Four months later I also realized that the pain in the joints in my hands had disappeared. I was delighted in this and did not expect my joints to return to their normal shape. However, 2 years after being on consistent pellet implantations I realized all the joints in my fingers had returned to normal shape and size. I was equally thrilled to realize that this condition was not an inevitable outcome of growing old; it was only that my body needed estradiol and testosterone in order for the joints to stay healthy.

After using the pellets for 18 years, Dr. Sun convinced me to increase my testosterone dosage even though was high out of range for normal for women. I am so thankful she understood this, as the increased dosage finally restored my sexual response to what it was before surgery. Up until that time, the pellet dose had brought the response back to 80 percent. I did not think to question it, as I was thrilled to feel anything, as I did not without the pellet implants. Now, 20 years of almost consistent pellet implants makes me a believer in them, and has given me the understanding that we women do not have to suffer with what we have thought were inevitable conditions of growing old. These conditions arise out of our loss of estradiol at menopause and for those of us who have had the misfortune of having our ovaries removed, the loss of testosterone also. I know when my pellets are running out. I marvel at how the body knows better than we do what it needs to maintain proper functioning. When my pellets start running low, I start in with problems with my memory and my ability to put thoughts together cohesively. I also start getting vertigo and become incontinent. Hot flashes can start and I start becoming more emotional and depressed, as well as start in sleeping less and sometimes have night sweats. In addition, I have found that when my body is stressed, because it utilizes them at a much greater rate, I need to have the implantations more often.

The difference in my quality of life is so profound that I know that I do not ever want to function again in my life without having these precious vitally important hormones replaced about every 4 months. I celebrate the doctors who utilized them in the beginning and all the doctors who have been open to realizing that pellets are a Godsend for women who do not absorb hormones readily and need them in order to function on a daily basis.

Elizabeth's story is not unusual. Many women have the same story. This is the worst situation that can occur when women who are already suffering from adrenal fatigue suddenly become surgically menopausal. These women develop severe menopausal symptoms, even to the point of suicidal depression and have difficulty carrying out daily activities. Many women have gone from doctor to doctor seeking help, only to be put on antidepressants, sleeping pills and all kinds of less effective hormone therapies that bring no relief. As previously observed and supported by research, subcutaneously implanted bio-identical hormone therapy is optimally effective and should be offered as a first-line therapy to avoid suffering and deterioration of health. Unfortunately, a good majority of gynecologists are unfamiliar with pellet therapy and, therefore, patients are not offered this option.

2. Women who have had a hysterectomy and/or oophorectomy, especially women younger than 45 years old.

Erica's story:

My name is Erica; I am 52 years old. When I was 16, I became pregnant for the first time and I had drastic mood swings. By the time I was in my 20s, I was one of those women who could kill somebody at that time of the month. For about 2 weeks each month, I was like that. I don't know how my husband stayed with me because I was horrible. At age 31, after having three children, I had to have a hysterectomy. When I awoke the next morning, I thought the room was excessively hot. The nurse told me that I was probably having hot flashes. I was immediately thrown into menopause, even though I still had my ovaries. I talked with the doctor about the hot flashes and he suggested that I use hormones. After a few different treatments without help, he told me about bio-identical hormone pellets. I was desperate and he put in the hormone implant. Within four to five days, I noticed a big difference in my life. My mood was even and my sex drive came back, which I had lost after the hysterectomy. My concentration was better. My doctor told me that the pellets help your bones and skin. I continued to get those implants. I'm now 52 and I've been getting the pellets well over 20 years. I have ten times more energy than other women my age. And I have an excitement about life. The pellets help me to keep evenly keeled and to think straight. I no longer have huge emotional dips. If a woman starts talking about symptoms of menopause, and her husband says that his wife has turned into a witch overnight, I tell them about the implants. They have told me that I have saved their marriages. The implants are my life, literally. If I don't have them, I know I won't have any quality of life.

3. **Menopausal women who are symptomatic and have not responded to other treatments.**

4. **Women who are perimenopausal and experience hormone fluctuations and are symptomatic with moodiness, inability to concentrate, hot flashes, weight gain or fatigue.**

5. **Women who have low testosterone and low libido.**

6. **Women who have hormone-related migraine headaches.**

7. **Women who are suffering from poor short-term memory and loss of multi-tasking skills.**

8. **Women who developed osteopenia or osteoporosis before 60 years old.**

9. **Postmenopausal women who want to achieve the best results from hormone replacement therapy to help prevent dementia, osteoporosis, or slow down the aging process.**

Breast Cancer and Hormone Therapy

Susan's story:

I am Susan, 59 years old, and a survivor of breast cancer. I was only 38 when diagnosed with breast cancer. I had a mastectomy; in fact, I had three surgeries in a year and a half. I also went into early menopause during that time. I suppose that being reproductive was something that Mother Nature thought was not in my best interest any more. I suffered for a long time without hormone replacement therapy because no doctors wanted to risk my having cancer again. My life became so sad. I could not sleep, and lost the ability to have good focus and to concentrate. My doctor told me that I had the hormone levels of a woman in her 80s. This scared me. I looked older than my years. I had osteopenia (loss of bone density that is considered a precursor to osteoporosis) and vaginal atrophy to a serious degree. My husband and I had not been active sexually for over seven years. It was pretty devastating for me.

I became so depressed that I seriously considered suicide. I literally felt every morning like I was pretty much dead anyway. It seemed as if my feet were already in the grave. Then I met Dr. Tutera in Arizona, who did the initial recommendation for insertion of pellets. The pellets have changed my life so much. My husband and I are active again. The cellular structure of my skin all over my body and in my vaginal area is much thicker. I am alert and astute. Since I had gone through early menopause and had lost my sex drive, I felt as if I was not a sexy person anymore. But after getting the pellets, I have started taking belly dancing and I feel very sensual and sexual again. This has been a remarkable turnaround. I am so very lucky to be alive and have this therapy available to me. It took a long time to find a doctor who was willing to give hormone replacement therapy to me. In fact, Dr. Tutera's patients have fewer incidences of all kinds of cancer than the general population. By maintaining healthy levels of hormones, the body can better deal with cancer cells. It is wonderful to be a happy, vibrant, and productive member of society. Since starting the pellets, I have earned my broker's license and started my own real estate company.

Fifty years ago, one in every 20 women was diagnosed with breast cancer; now it is one in every six or seven. Birth control pills and hormone replacement therapy have been named as the culprits for this dramatic change in statistics. Similarly, consider the rate of prostate cancer in men. It was also one in 20 only 50 years ago and is now one in every five men, just as with women. But men, unlike women, have not been receiving hormone replacement as routinely as women. So, if hormone replacement is the cause for the increase of breast cancer in women, what is the explanation for the increase of prostate cancer in men? Part of the explanation is that both sexes are living appreciably longer, and that these cancers increase in frequency with age. Also both men and women are now being examined more routinely than at any other time and this will increase the number of cancers found. Fifty years ago, there were no such things as mammograms and PSA exams.

Another part of the answer can be found by looking at other factors. First, there are many chemicals and toxins in the environment that people did not have to contend with 50 years ago. Many of these chemicals and toxins are carcinogens (cancer causing) or hormone imposters, which means they are not actually hormones but can stimulate hormone receptors and cause unwanted results in the body. Another factor is that we are so much more stressed today with a fast-paced lifestyle that is inundated by wireless technology, loud music, and nonstop noise. Higher levels of stress lower our immunity. When immunity is reduced, cancer and other illnesses occur at increased rates.

As we discussed in the previous chapter, bio-identical estrogen replacement therapy with pellets, balanced with bio-identical progesterone and testosterone does not increase the breast cancer rate, not even for women already diagnosed with breast cancer after cancer treatment.

Dr. Tutera studied 976 women on bio-identical hormone pellet therapy over a period of ten years and found only one woman who developed breast cancer.[41] His research suggests a much lower incidence of cancer among women on bio-identical hormone replacement therapy delivered via subcutaneously implanted pellets than occurs in the general population.

Davelaar, who studied 267 women for twenty-five years, found that women using estradiol pellets had less cancer of the breast than a control group that received no hormone treatment.[34]

Most women develop breast cancer when they are menopausal, the premenopausal ones usually become menopausal after chemotherapy or radiation for breast cancer. Many of them suffer tremendously with menopausal symptoms, especially from depression, fatigue and low libido. Scared by the possibility of recurrence of breast cancer and warnings from their physicians, they suffer silently without seeking treatment.

This suffering is needless. There is enough scientific evidence that proper hormone treatment improves the quality of life and boosts the immune system, and thus does not increase the likelihood of a recurrence of cancer.

Breast Cancer Prevention

Breast cancer is one of the most common cancers in females. The older you are, the higher the rate of breast cancer. Breast cancer has a lot to do with environmental toxins, especially xenohormones (chemicals that mimic the effect of estrogen, and cause DNA mutations).

There are ways to reduce breast cancer:

1. **Reduce Exposure to Environmental Toxins**

   Hormones are injected into animals. Thus the meat of beef, pork and chicken, as well as their products such as milk, cheese and eggs contain the injected hormones. Make sure to buy organic meats and produce to avoid exposure to these xenohormones. Also, reduce your exposure to pesticides, plastics and other industrial by-products. Please see pages 166-167 for details.

2. **Improve Detoxification**

   It is important to detoxify the estrogen that is in our bodies once it has performed its vital functions, as the longer it stays in the body, the greater the risk it can lead to estrogen dominance or breast cancer. Once estrogen is detoxified, it can be processed for elimination.

   There are several ways to improve estrogen detoxification:

   - Diet: Diets high in cruciferous vegetables such as broccoli, cauliflower, cabbage and sprouts can increase the C-2 hydroxylation pathway.

- Supplements: Intake of nutrients involved in liver Phase I and Phase II detoxification pathways, including vitamins A, B6, B12, C, folate, magnesium, zinc, selenium, glycine, taurine, glutamine, cysteine and methionine.

- Probiotics: Probiotics, which are healthy intestinal bacteria, can reduce the harmful bacteria that may interfere with estrogen excretion.

- Fiber can improve elimination.

- Evening Primrose Oil, 1000 mg daily, helps to reduce inflammation of the breast tissue.

3. Improve Your Immunity

- Proper nutrition, focus on a diet that reduces inflammation. Please see page 132 for details.

- Make sleep a priority. See pages 264-266 for details.

- Stress reduction and coping skills. See pages 267-270 for details.

- Regular exercise. See pages 271-273 for details.

4. Balance Hormones

- Balance estrogen with testosterone and progesterone if needed.

- Optimize good hormones such as melatonin, DHEA, thyroid hormone and growth hormone (HGH).

- Reduce harmful hormones such as insulin and cortisol.

As discussed previously, hormone balance protects the breast cells. These methods not only protect us from breast cancer, they also reduce estrogen dominance related conditions such as fibrocystic breast disease, premenstrual tension, heavy menstrual bleeding and fibroid tumors.

HRT and Menopausal Women

It is not a given that all menopausal women need bio-identical hormone replacement therapy, but nearly everyone can benefit from it.

If you are menopausal and have good adrenal function, a healthy, stress-free lifestyle, no family history of diabetes, hypertension, osteoporosis, senile dementia and no menopausal symptoms, you may choose not to use any hormone replacement therapy. Remember, bio-identical hormone replacement therapy reduces cardiovascular diseases, Alzheimer's disease, dementia, osteoporosis, and muscle loss.

The misconception is if your hot flashes are gone, a woman is finished with menopause, whereas in truth starting into menopause is the first step towards aging and dying. The problem is that degenerative diseases such as osteoporosis, memory loss, atherosclerosis, fatigue, decreased immunity and arthritis do not come all at once—they progress gradually and often imperceptibly until their presence is too painful or obvious to ignore. Keeping sex hormones in the younger-age range, combined with a healthy lifestyle, can slow down or prevent these aging-related diseases.

As an internist, I have seen many women in their 70s and 80s who had already developed osteoporosis, dementia, urinary incontinence and cardiovascular diseases. By this time, their conditions have become very difficult to treat. But even at this stage, their quality of life can be better with bio-identical hormone pellet therapy. My oldest patient on pellets is an 88-year-old woman who, after one year of treatment, feels that pellet therapy has helped her memory, sleep pattern and energy levels. She wants to continue this therapy for the quality of life it gives her.

Laboratory Testing for Hormones

In order to implant the correct dosage of pellets, the body's baseline hormone levels need to be established. These can be determined by blood tests. Several blood tests are involved in evaluating hormone functions. First and most foremost is FSH (follicular stimulating hormone). This hormone is secreted by the pituitary gland in the brain, which is the master regulator of the hormone systems. FSH regulates estrogen. If the body needs estrogen, FSH rises to stimulate the ovaries to produce more estrogen. If the body has enough estrogen, FSH decreases since it does not need to stimulate the ovaries to produce more estrogen.

Before menopause, FSH is typically below 10. After menopause, it is between 25 and 120. The higher the FSH, the more the body needs estrogen. Most women do not feel good if their FSH levels are over 50. At a perimenopausal stage, when women are still having periods, FSH can be unreliable—both high and low—if the samples were obtained at different times because as estrogen declines, the FSH rises, which stimulates the ovaries to produce more estrogen. Then FSH declines, which leads to reduced estrogen. At this stage many women are symptomatic with hot flashes, night sweats, irregular periods or mood swings due to fluctuations of their hormone levels. Yet if they only examine blood tests, their doctors may well tell them that they are fine, and not menopausal, as some women have hormone deficient symptoms even when their laboratory tests show their hormone levels to be within normal ranges.

Other hormones I check are estradiol, progesterone, and testosterone, both total and free levels. I also check SHBG (sex hormone binding globulin). A higher SHBG indicates that the level of free hormones is lower and symptoms are more likely to occur.

For adrenal function, I check cortisol and DHEA (hormones secreted by adrenal glands) in the morning. The blood tests for adrenal functions are not that reliable and need to be interpreted with the patient's symptoms. If I see that cortisol is very high or very low, it confirms my diagnosis of adrenal stress or exhaustion.

Most of the time, I see normal cortisol and low DHEA, which indicates that the patient is in some degree of adrenal fatigue. At this stage, the adrenal glands are still functioning, but the production of DHEA has been lowered to conserve the adrenal glands.

I also check thyroid functions by monitoring TSH, free T3, and free T4. I always check thyroid hormones and adrenal hormones because they are so intimately related to the sex hormones. Just like an orchestra, many players are involved and they have to play together harmoniously. With hormone replacement therapy, we need to pay attention to all the hormones, especially the major players of the sex, adrenal, and thyroid hormones as people feel their best and will be their healthiest when their hormones are balanced.

Side Effects of Pellets Therapy

Side effects of pellet therapy are few, and at best rare, if done by well trained and experienced physicians. The insertion procedure on occasion may cause the possibility of slight pain, bleeding and infection of the incision site. There may be transient breast tenderness and water retention (ankle swelling) that disappears quickly and usually only occurs with the first insertion.

The real issue is proper dosage of hormone pellets. If the dosage is too low, a person will not feel much improvement. If the dosage is too high, there may be side effects. For instance, if estradiol is too high a woman can develop breast soreness, retain water, or gain fat. If testosterone is too high, individuals can become more aggressive or preoccupied with sexual thoughts; and acne or facial hair can develop. This may also lead to male pattern baldness in the long-term. Again, this is where we advise you see a well-trained and experienced physician.

Another problem is spotting or menstruation, which is usually the result of insufficient progesterone to balance estrogen's growth effect on the lining of the uterus. This most commonly occurs because a patient does not take progesterone correctly. It can also be due to fibroid tumors, endometrial polyps and in rare instances endometrial cancer. If bleeding persists after increasing the dosage of progesterone, a pelvic ultrasound is required, along with an endometrial biopsy.

It is a good idea to start conservatively when it comes to pellet dosage. It is easy to add more pellets but it is very difficult to remove the pellets after implantation. The pellet dosage also needs to be adjusted periodically according to each individual's response to achieve optimal results.

Contraindications for Pellet Therapy

There are certain conditions that must be considered when determining if pellet therapy is suitable for someone. It is not advisable to give pellet therapy to persons with the following conditions.

1. Untreated breast, uterine or ovarian cancer. For women who have finished their breast cancer treatment and exhibit no evidence of residual cancer, I do offer testosterone, with or without a very small dose of estradiol, if they want to receive pellet therapy. This also applies to women who have had their uterus or ovaries removed due to cancer and who exhibit no evidence of residual cancer. I will not administer treatment if the patient or I have any doubts.

2. History of fibroid tumors. Since estrogen may cause growth of fibroids, estrogen doses have to be modified to a lower level to prevent bleeding. Dr. Tutera and I recommend that women with large fibroids have them treated first by surgery or uterine artery embolization before starting therapy.

3. History of multiple chemical sensitivities or leaky gut syndrome can have adverse effects due to the already toxin overload. In these cases I help detoxify these patients first. Once this is accomplished we can begin using pellet therapy, although more cautiously and with reduced dosage.

Self-assessment for Estrogen Dominance and PMS

Considering their importance to our health and well-being, it is crucial that our hormones exist in a state of balance. To help gauge your current state of hormonal balance, take a moment to consider the following questions.

1. Do you have heavy menstrual bleeding?

2. Do you have breast tenderness before your period?

3. Do you have fibrocystic breast disease or a uterine fibroid tumor?

4. Do you have mood swings, anxiety, or depression before your period?

5. Do you have water retention or do you feel bloated?

6. Do you have migraine headaches associated with your menstrual cycle?

If you answered "*yes*" to more than one question, you probably have estrogen dominance, which is an imbalance between estrogen and progesterone.

Self-assessment for Testosterone Deficiency

As we have seen, testosterone also plays a very important role in women's health. Consider the following questions to gain a better idea of where your levels of testosterone currently stand.

1. Do you have low libido?

2. Do you experience mental fogginess or have difficulty concentrating?

3. Do you feel depressed or anxious?

4. Do you feel fatigued or lack interest in doing things?

5. Are you losing muscle tone or is it hard to build muscle mass even with exercise?

6. Are you gaining fat in your abdominal area?

7. Do you have dry skin? Are you experiencing vaginal dryness?

8. Do you have migraine headaches?

If you answered "*yes*" to more than two questions, you probably have testosterone deficiency.

Points to Remember

1. Bio-identical hormone replacement therapy, if done right, does not increase the risk of breast cancer.

2. Subcutaneously implanted hormones in the pellet form is the most physiological route of delivery, and they achieve the best results in terms of minimizing menopausal symptoms.

3. It is important to replace and balance deficient sex hormones because the benefits go beyond reducing menopausal symptoms. Proper hormone balance actually prevents age related diseases and slows down the aging process.

4. Hormone replacement therapy has to be individualized and monitored to achieve the best results and to reduce or eliminate side effects.

5. Testosterone deficiency in women is a neglected problem that can occur even in young women.

6. Adrenal fatigue is very common. Menopause makes adrenal fatigue worse and vice versa.

7. Thyroid, adrenal, and sex hormones are interrelated. Replacing one can affect the others. They must all be monitored and treated together, as needed, to stay in harmonious balance and optimize optimal health.

CHAPTER 5

Male Testosterone Deficiency

There is no doubt that hormones play a significant role in women's health. The life enhancing benefits of bio-identical hormone therapy that were discussed last chapter—physical vitality, emotional balance, disease prevention and the slowing down of the aging process—continue to be documented by medical studies and confirmed by the patient success stories we witness in our practices every day. But did you know that men can also stand to benefit greatly from bio-identical hormone therapy? This is true—more men than ever are becoming aware of the detrimental effects of hormone loss on their bodies and the potential of pellet therapy to restore their former robustness and zest for life. While it is true that hormones like testosterone exist in much higher amounts in men, the gradual decline of this vital hormone causes just as many problems for men as the loss of estrogen does in women. For instance, take my patient Lee and the many difficulties he faced when his levels of testosterone declined dangerously low.

Lee's story:

I am Lee, aged 63. A decade ago I was CEO of a public health care company when a hereditary iron metabolism disease, hemochromatosis, forced my retirement. With iron-poisoned organs, my convalescence took years. Dedicated exercise helped, but I was hampered with vital organ scar tissue, and I was forced into having a pint of blood drained every two months for the rest of my life to remove excess iron build-up. Since my testicles were damaged and my libido had suffered, I asked my doctor for testosterone injections. Even though my blood levels were very low, he declined, saying that it was just something I would have to live with. So, I did, year upon year out of "unnecessary" necessity, I wrote off most of my sex life. What a void. What a waste. What a tragedy. Totally unnecessary!

Then, I heard about bio-identical hormone replacement therapy, which led me to a highly trained, board-certified internal medicine specialist, Karen Sun, M.D., in Irvine, California. She was wonderful, a real and totally dedicated doctor who immediately seized upon my chronic panoply of male hormone-deficient symptoms of fatigue, insomnia, anxiety, depression, "feeling old," and of course, a minimal sex drive. Fresh blood tests proved that my free testosterone levels were next to zero. Dr. Sun quickly initiated "just under the skin" hormone replacement pellets, a cinchy, painless, 15 minute procedure. She closely monitored my astonishing rebirth thereafter.

Within weeks I felt 10, maybe 20 years younger. I slept well and, at long last, woke up every morning refreshed and free of cobwebs. I acquired zest, which lasted all day. My anxiety and depression dissipated, and I became hungry for love. Although the hormones increased my appetite, I thwarted weight gain by increasing my exercise, which I suddenly had the energy to accomplish.

Testosterone has been used successfully for years to treat men with abnormally low testosterone levels, a medical condition called male hypogonadism. In most men, testosterone secretion starts to decline at the rate of one to three percent a year after age 30. This means that by age 50, a man may have lost 20 to 60 percent of his testosterone production. By the age of 70, 70 percent of all men fit into the criteria of hypogonadism. The marked decline in energy levels, mental focus, libido and emotional stability that accompanies this process has become so common and widespread that a new term, "andropause," has been coined to describe the transition men undergo when hormone levels bottom out. Andropause, like menopause, is due to the decline of testosterone but, unlike women who experience a sudden drop of hormones, it occurs gradually and the symptoms are less dramatic.

Symptoms of Andropause and Testosterone Deficiency

Decreased energy, fatigue.

Reduced muscle strength and mass, less exercise endurance, and prolonged recovery from exercise.

Decreased cognitive function, such as poor memory or lack of mental sharpness.

Less sexual interest and/or performance.
Loss of interest; crabby, depressed mood.
Weight gain, particularly fat around the midsection.
Insomnia, decreased quality of sleep.
Thinning of body hair and dry skin.
Joint pain.
Osteoporosis or decreased bone density (X-ray finding).

Diagnosis of Testosterone Deficiency

1. Blood test for both total and free testosterone level:

Most testosterone binds with SHBG (sex hormone binding globulin) and is not active. Like a car in a car carrier, it's not driving on the road. Only free testosterone, testosterone that is not bound with SHBG, is small enough to enter the body's cells and work. The production of total testosterone decreases with age, but the SHBG remains the same. This leads to a reduced amount of free testosterone and consequently of the functions testosterone provides. To determine the amount of testosterone available to perform in the body, it is important to check both total testosterone and free testosterone.

2. Blood test for estradiol level:

Aging also causes a testosterone-estrogen imbalance in men. Specifically, reduced free testosterone with the same or increased estrogen changes the ratio of testosterone to estrogen. A testosterone-estrogen imbalance can cause many diseases associated with aging, including heart attack, stroke, and prostate hypertrophy (enlargement).

Common Reasons for Testosterone-estrogen Imbalance

- Liver dysfunction. As the body's major detoxification organ, the liver eliminates excess estrogen and sex hormone-binding protein. The liver can have reduced function due to the effects of alcohol, drugs, infection, heart failure, aging, or liver diseases, which leads to increased estrogen and sex hormone-binding protein.

- Obesity. Fat cells, especially around the abdominal area, secrete estrogen and aromatase, which is an enzyme that converts testosterone to estrogen. Increased estrogen in men further increases abdominal fat. This becomes a vicious cycle!

- Nutritional deficiency, especially zinc, which is a natural aromatase inhibitor, will make things worse.

Testosterone and the Prostate Gland

Many people, including doctors, think prostate cancer is linked to testosterone. This is the most common reason that men shy away from testosterone replacement therapy. Most published scientific papers however, suggest otherwise.[42,43] Estrogens, especially the environmental xenohormones, not testosterone, are more to blame.

Living longer contribute to the increase in the incidence of cancers, especially prostate cancer. Additionally, 50 years ago there were not as many chemicals and toxins in the environment to disrupt the body's hormone systems. Now we have so many more toxins, especially xenoestrogens, from certain foods, pesticides and plastics. These are aggravating factors that I see contributing to the cause of the increase of cancers in the reproductive systems of both men and women.

If prostate cancer cells are present, however, increasing the level of testosterone will speed the growth of cancer. This is why the PSA (prostate specific antigen) blood level should be checked before and after testosterone treatment.

For men who have prostate hypertrophy (enlargement), testosterone treatment can increase the size of the prostate even more by its conversion to DHT (dihydrotestosterone) and estradiol, both of which can stimulate prostate growth. Proscar (a prescription medicine) reduces DHT and Aromasin (a prescription medicine) is an aromatase inhibitor that can reduce the conversion of testosterone to estrogen. Both medications can be used to prevent or slow down prostate growth.

Saw palmetto is a supplement that can reduce DHT formation. It also inhibits the binding of estrogen to prostate cells and the binding of DHT to the prostate gland. Saw palmetto reduces inflammation of the prostate and relaxes the sphincter tone around the urethra so that the flow of urine can improve. For these reasons, saw palmetto has become a very popular prostate supplement for men. Another popular supplement is chrysin, which is derived from the plant Passiflora caerulea. It works as a natural aromatase inhibitor. It is also a potent antioxidant and has the added benefit of reducing inflammation. Formulas that combine all the protective herbal agents, such as saw palmetto, lycopene, chrysin, and zinc are recommended for prostate health.

Testosterone and Depression

Have you ever encountered a grumpy old man? You do not have to grow old to be grumpy, but there certainly are a lot of grumpy men who are old. There is a hormonal reason for that too.

Published studies show that HRT increases the sense of well-being in andropausal men.[44] Studies also show that a low level of testosterone is associated with anxiety, depression, irritability and other psychological disorders in andropausal men. An article in the *American Journal of Geriatric Psychiatry* reviewed studies published from 1966 to 1999 to determine if there was a moderate decline of total testosterone and, more significantly, a decline of bioavailable (free) testosterone in aging males.[45] The article's survey revealed some interesting findings. Elderly males who were depressed appeared to have the lowest testosterone levels. In males with normal testosterone levels, HRT did not have a significant effect on mood. However, in treating depressed men with low testosterone levels, HRT was shown to be very effective. This article advocated HRT as a primary or adjunct treatment of depression in elderly males. Another article showed that testosterone replacement therapy is more effective than antidepressants in men with lower testosterone levels.[46]

Testosterone and the Cardiovascular System

A recent study published in the *Journal of American College of Cardiology* shows that testosterone helps to protect men from atherosclerosis (hardening of the arteries).[47] They performed ultrasound testing on aging men to assess the thickness of the carotid artery, the artery that supplies blood to the brain. As the testosterone level dropped the artery wall thickness increased, which impairs delivery of oxygen to the brain. The result can be dementia and strokes.

Testosterone helps to build muscles, including heart muscles.[48] Testosterone also dilates coronary arteries, reduces heart attacks, reduces high blood pressure, and helps to lower cholesterol levels.[49,50]

Testosterone causes an erection by dilating blood vessels in the penis due to stimulating the production of nitrous oxide. The same effect also happens in coronary arteries. The most abundant receptor sites found for testosterone are not in the penis or the brain, but are located in the coronary blood vessels.

If you have high blood pressure or cardiovascular disease, you should check your free testosterone and estrogen levels. Treating testosterone deficiency and improving the testosterone/estrogen ratio may be one of the most effective and natural ways to treat cardiovascular diseases.

Testosterone and Insulin—Diabetes

Stephen's story:

I am Stephen, in my mid 50s. I had been a very healthy, energetic, active business professional until in my early 40s, when I started feeling somewhat "off." My weight gradually increased by 20 pounds, which was somewhat disconcerting. I just didn't feel right. Then, after I visited a marshmallow factory in Las Vegas and tried some samples, I started to feel terrible on the drive back to California. Normally, I could drive long distances with no problem. But on this drive, I didn't even make it to the state line. I had to ask my wife, Debby, to drive. That had never happened before. Then I passed out and woke up hours later in Newport Beach. It turns out that I was in a diabetic coma. That was the cornerstone of my health problems, which led to my seeing a very reputable internist.

Every time I mentioned a problem to my internist, he gave me a prescription for it. But I was feeling worse as the years went by. Indeed, the more medicine he gave me, the worse I felt. And, always, my doctor's answer to my every health question was: "Well, you are getting older.

You're going to have some pain with one thing or another." None of this made sense to me. So, I started asking around and doing research. That is when I learned about hormones in general, and specifically, as a guy I was focusing on testosterone. I asked my internist about my testosterone levels and just got his typical answer about getting older. Then he gave me another prescription for something completely unrelated.

I pushed my internist to test my testosterone level. A man's testosterone should be at 1,000; mine was 93. A couple of things don't work well at a T level of 93. Not only that, the little blue pill (Viagra) did not work for me and that really concerned me. So, I went on a mission to learn everything that I could about hormone replacement. I have followed Suzanne Somers and her books on the subject.

Then, I found Karen Sun, M.D. through a couple who are friends of ours. At a dinner at their home, I noticed that the wife had more energy than usual, and I asked if she happened to be on bio-identical hormones, not a typical conversation for us. But I had been doing research and thought I would discuss it with her. She confirmed that was true and then explained how Dr. Sun had done the procedure to implant pellets about the size of grains of rice. She added that her general overall feeling was now just fantastic. I told her, "You are a sign from heaven."

So, I went to see Dr. Sun and she spent more time counseling me in our first session than the years of visits that I had spent with my internist, collectively. She took blood tests and gave me information that my other doctor never talked about with me. She also told me that she thought we could get me off most of the medications I was taking. Two days after she gave me the pellets I felt like I was in my early 30s again. Within five days, every ache in my body was gone.

Since I have been on the pellets, I have lost nearly 30 pounds, and that is without doing anything special to lose weight. I just feel great now, and we have managed to eliminate most of my meds. Also, emotionally I had been experiencing a high level of edginess and things would set me off more quickly before I was on the pellets. I was not quite as patient, but with the pellets, my emotions are very much in check. I am a touchy-feely type of person, and when the romantic part of my life dropped to almost zero, I was not happy. I did not want to hang up that saddle for the rest of my life. Ever since I've been "pelletized," that area has come roaring back. I feel great!

Studies have linked low levels of testosterone with diabetes.[51,52] Testosterone replacement therapy reduces insulin resistance.[51] Dhindsa et al. showed that a third of men with type II diabetes have low free testosterone levels.[53] A low level of testosterone causes low lean muscle mass and higher abdominal fat, which leads to insulin resistance and increased risk for cardiovascular diseases. Testosterone replacement reduces body fat, increases lean muscle and improves strength.[53] Many diabetic men who have low testosterone suffer from depression, poor memory, insomnia, fatigue, low bone density, heart disease and erectile dysfunction. In Steven's case, he was able to lose weight, lower his blood pressure and diabetic medication after the pellet treatment. Most importantly, his life is back!

Testosterone therapy should be incorporated into treatment plans for diabetic patients with low testosterone levels and may well be one of the most effective and natural treatments available.

Testosterone and Alzheimer's Disease

Research is revealing a strong link between testosterone levels and Alzheimer's disease. One study shows that longitudinal assessment of serum free testosterone concentration predicts memory performance and cognitive status in elderly men.[54] Another study also supports that testosterone replacement reduces the risk of Alzheimer's disease by preventing the production of beta-amyloid protein.[55]

In my practice, I routinely observe that mood and mental sharpness in patients improves after testosterone replacement therapy. This is the most common reason my patients want to continue the treatment. They not only appreciate the benefits of an improved libido, they also welcome the mental sharpness and enhanced sense of well-being that accompanies testosterone therapy.

Testosterone and Osteoporosis

According to the National Osteoporosis Foundation, 2 million men in the U.S. have osteoporosis and another 3 million are at risk. Gradual decline of testosterone (T) is the most common reason for osteoporosis in aging men. In one study, 59 percent of men with hip fractures had low T, compared with 18 percent of men in the control group.[56] Fractures occur at a later age in men than in women because men's bones are denser than women's. Testosterone receptors are present in osteoblasts (bone-forming cells), and many studies report the beneficial effects of testosterone treatment in older men, showing an increase in bone mineral density and a slowing of bone degeneration.

For men affected by osteoporosis, getting testosterone replacement therapy may work better than taking prescription medications, with the added plus of providing a wide variety of benefits such as enhanced energy, emotional balance, mental clarity and revitalized libido.

Is Testosterone Replacement Therapy the Answer for Aging Men?

Do you want to increase your muscle mass, strengthen your bones, improve your cardiovascular system, boost your mood, sharpen your memory, charge up your libido and improve your energy? To men suffering from the ill-effects of hormone loss and age-related diseases, these things may very well sound like key ingredients to the fountain of youth.

Yet far from being a fantasy, treatment with bio-identical testosterone pellets can be a very real part of men's lives, bringing benefits that enhance the quality of their lives tremendously. According to the statistics, men everywhere are standing up and taking notice. HRT in aging men is growing in popularity. According to IMS Health, a company that tracks pharmaceutical sales, 2.4 million testosterone prescriptions were filled in 2004, more than twice the number that were filled in 2000. The questions arise: Is testosterone safe? What is the down side? So far, no long-term human study has been done, but we can borrow what we have learned from hormone replacement therapy for women. In general, the rules should be the same.

Testosterone—Routes of Delivery

1. Intramuscular Injection

An intramuscular injection is given every two weeks and results in fluctuating hormone levels. This is not time-released, low-dosage pellet therapy. Also, the drugs available for injections are not bio-identical testosterone; Depo-Testosterone (testosterone cypionate) and methyltestosterone are commonly used.

2. Transdermal: Patch, Cream, or Gel

Androderm patch is available by prescription. The patch needs to be changed daily and skin irritation can be a problem. AndroGel is also available by prescription. The gel or cream can be rubbed into the skin on the lower abdomen, upper arm, or shoulder area. It causes less skin irritation than the patch. Users must avoid showering or bathing for several hours after application to ensure adequate absorption. A potential side effect is the possibility of transferring the testosterone to your partner. The absorption rate may vary resulting in an insignificant improvement of the testosterone level, especially if a man has a very low testosterone level at the beginning of treatment.

3. Oral

The oral form of delivery is not a recommended route. Due to processing through the liver, taking testosterone orally may cause an unfavorable cholesterol profile, and an increase in the risk of blood clots along with possible liver damage.

4. Sublingual (under the tongue)

The sublingual route allows the testosterone to be absorbed directly into the bloodstream. It becomes oral, however, if it is swallowed before it dissolves and absorbed. It can also cause gum irritation and may have an unpleasant taste. The sublingual route causes a surge of testosterone, which lasts 10-12 hours, and it needs to be used twice a day.

5. Pellet Implants

Bio-identical hormones pellet implants are placed subcutaneously just under the skin. These hormones are released into the bloodstream slowly and last between four to six months. Since it bypasses the liver, this is by far thc most physiological and effective delivery system of the right hormones in the proper dosage that attains a steady blood level all of the time.

In my practice, I have seen many men who have tried testosterone in the form of gels, patches or shots, but did not achieve the results they wanted, whereas subcutaneously implanted pellets have worked well for them. Plus, pellets are a very easy system of administration. There is no gel, cream, or patch to apply every day; just a simple procedure performed every four to six months.

Rules of Testosterone Replacement

Just as with women's hormone replacement, there are special rules to observe when utilizing testosterone therapy in men.

1. Only replace testosterone when it is at a low functional level for that patient.

2. Use bio-identical hormones.

3. Monitor the hormone levels; be sure they are in a normal range and maintain a proper testosterone to estrogen ratio.

4. Use the most physiological route of delivery, which is either transdermal or subcutaneous pellet implants.

5. Monitor the PSA level to make sure it does not increase with the hormone treatment.

Indications for Testosterone Replacement

The following symptoms may indicate that your testosterone levels are low.

Depression, crabby mood, or loss of interest in activities.
Fatigue or low energy level.
Low libido or erectile dysfunction.

Poor memory, lack of concentration, or mental fog.
Reduced muscle mass and/or exercise endurance.
Osteoporosis or osteopenia.
Diabetes, hypertension and cardiovascular diseases.
Insomnia or poor quality of sleep.
Weight gain, especially fat around the middle.

Side Effects of Testosterone Replacement

When considering the possibility of side effects in testosterone replacement therapy, it is important to remember that the side effects of HRT are related to super-high dosages, not to the proper levels that are created by bio-identical hormones in pellet therapy. Such high levels of testosterone can:

Increase bone marrow production of red blood cells, which leads to an increase in blood volume and blood pressure, and an increased risk of blood clots.
Cause acne.
Lead to testicular shrinkage (atrophy).
Increase prostate hypertrophy (enlargement).
Stimulate the growth of prostate cancer if it is already present.
Enlarge breasts, if too much testosterone is converted to estrogen.
Aggravate sleep apnea.
Cause male pattern baldness.

Contraindications for Testosterone Replacement

There are instances when testosterone replacement therapy should not be considered. Do not use when there is either:

1. Untreated prostate cancer or breast cancer (rare but can occur in men).

2. Untreated benign prostate hypertrophy (BPH).

Points to Remember

1. Testosterone production declines with age. By the age of 70, 70 percent of men have testosterone deficiency.

2. Testosterone replacement therapy is not solely meant to boost the libido. It improves mood and memory, builds muscle and bone density, reduces body fat and helps to prevent or treat hypertension, diabetes and cardiovascular diseases associated with testosterone deficiency.

3. Use bio-identical hormones and a physiological route of delivery such as gel, patch or subcutaneously implanted pellets if you decide to do testosterone replacement therapy. Pellet implants are the easiest and most effective treatment method. Consider trying pellet therapy if use of the patch, cream or gel does not produce the results you desire.

4. Patients' free and total testosterone levels should always be monitored: higher than normal hormone levels may lead to side effects and complications.

5. PSA levels should be monitored closely, especially in the first year of receiving testosterone treatment.

6. It is also important to monitor estradiol levels and the testosterone-to-estradiol ratio. The use of an aromatase inhibitor should be considered if estradiol is too high.

7. Nutritional supplements with antioxidants, minerals, vitamins C and E, lycopene, zinc, selenium, and herbs such as saw palmetto and chrysin are helpful for prostate health.

Since I began treating patients with bio-identical hormone pellets, more and more people have become attuned to the hormonal needs of their bodies. As the popularity of pellet therapy continues to grow, I find it particularly gratifying to know that increasing numbers of men as well as women are becoming aware of the vital, supportive role these wondrous pellets play in their lives.

The gradual onset of andropause in men can cause a great amount of suffering due to the loss of key hormones like testosterone. Yet, thanks to pellet therapy the conditions that many men once believed to be a natural and unavoidable part of growing older—sagging muscles, loss of libido, depression, anxiety, and a lack of energy—are no longer a mandatory part of the aging process. Through treatment that brings hormone levels back into balance, detrimental symptoms can be reversed, depleted systems can be restored to their once plentiful states, and men can once again enjoy the strength, vitality and zest for life that they have always enjoyed.

CHAPTER 6

Adrenal Fatigue—The Stress Epidemic

The adrenal glands secrete hormones to help the body cope with stress. About the size of a walnut, the adrenal glands sit on top of the kidneys and produce powerful hormones to sustain the entire body and its life processes. As a matter of fact, we would die without adrenal hormones.

Stress Factors

Stress assaults us every day. Relationships can be stressful due to, among other things, marital problems and divorce, death or illness of family members, or challenges with raising children. Our professional commitments involve such stressors as the need to work long hours, the hassles of commuting, troubles with coworkers, the pressures of deadlines and disliking current employment or needing to change jobs. When there is not enough money to pay the bills, the worry created can be quite traumatic. Conversely, having too much money can cause stress. Additionally, we can stress ourselves internally when we strive too hard to be perfect.

We can have physical stressors, too, such as surgery, malnutrition, colds or influenza, chronic insomnia, injuries, etc. Toxic chemicals in our environment and pollutants in the air also stress our bodies.

As these stressors creep into our lives, they can be debilitating and lead to problems with anxiety and depression. Chronic stress also leads to hypertension, diabetes, heart attack, stroke, cardiovascular disease, ulcers and other serious diseases. When people say, "The stress is killing me," they are closer to the truth than they realize. Stress can, and does, kill.

Chronic stress also places a strain on our adrenal glands, which over time leads to adrenal fatigue.

Adrenal Hormones and Their Actions

Adrenal Medulla

The adrenal medulla (inside part) secretes:

1. Epinephrine (adrenaline).

2. Norepinephrine.

These hormones trigger the body's response to the arousal to "fight or flight." They work on our autonomic (or automatic) nervous system, which increases our blood pressure and heart rate. They also cause muscle contractions.

In the GI (gastrointestinal) system, these hormones cause diarrhea or constipation, which, if chronic, can lead to irritable bowel syndrome. These hormones are also neurotransmitters that stimulate the brain. They put us on high alert if danger threatens. These are also the hormones that give us stage fright.

Adrenal Cortex

The adrenal cortex (outside part) produces several hormones:

1. DHEA and pregnenolone, the precursors to progesterone, testosterone and estrogen.

2. Cortisol (cortisone), which increases blood sugar. When our ancestors saw a tiger, they had to react right away in order to survive. The adrenal glands pump cortisol to increase the blood sugar as the source of energy for the body's ability to respond to extraordinary circumstances. Cortisol also regulates our immune response and reduces inflammation.

3. Aldosterone, a hormone that increases body fluids. It increases sodium retention and potassium excretion, leading to fluid retention and increased blood pressure.

Stages of Stress and Adrenal Fatigue

Stress wears down the adrenal glands over time. Hence, damage to the adrenals occurs gradually. The onset of adrenal fatigue is not sudden; rather, it occurs in three stages.

First Stage Adrenal Fatigue

The first stage is termed arousal and is referred to as adrenal hyperfunction. For example, if a person sees a house on fire, the adrenal glands release a spurt of adrenaline, which causes higher blood pressure, rapid heartbeat, greater alertness and more tense muscles. A slower surge of cortisol produces extra blood sugar so that individual can use the energy boost for the fight-or-flight response. When the emergency is gone, the body returns to normal.

Second Stage Adrenal Fatigue

The second stage of adrenal fatigue is called adaptation. Being in a chronically stressed environment is like living in a war zone. A person is prepared to fight at any time and, accordingly, sustains high levels of adrenal hormones that can change the body in several ways:

- Glucose (blood sugar) metabolism is harmfully altered. Elevated levels of cortisol increase blood sugar as a source of energy. If the body does not burn this sugar off, it will store the excess as fat. Higher sugar levels also stimulate insulin secretion from the pancreas. Eventually, cell membranes become insensitive to this increase in insulin, and the body has to secrete even more insulin to handle the sugar load. This is referred to as insulin resistance; chronic elevated cortisol levels lead to weight gain, diabetes, hypertension and cardiovascular diseases.

- The cardiovascular system is negatively impacted. Aldosterone by altering the sodium and potassium ratio increases blood volume and elevates blood pressure. Adrenaline also increases blood pressure.

- A high cortisol level reduces the transformation of thyroid hormone from T4 to the more active form of T3. This leads to subclinical hypothyroidism, which causes fatigue and further weight gain.

- High cortisol levels can affect our brain function negatively, impairing our memory, inducing brain fog, making tasks harder to handle and making it easy to become irritable.

- Reduced sex hormone production. Stress overworks the adrenal glands. The exhausted adrenals produce less DHEA the precursor of sex hormones. Before menopause, 30 percent of the sex hormones are generated by the adrenal glands and 70 percent by the ovaries. After menopause, the ratio reverses. Most of the sex hormones then must come from the adrenal glands, and if the tired adrenals cannot meet this demand due to chronic stress, the body will have a hard time dealing with menopause. Low levels of progesterone lead to estrogen dominance, which is due to too much estrogen and/or not enough progesterone. This can lead to PMS, excess menstrual bleeding, breast tenderness, or even fibrocystic disease or fibroid tumors. Low levels of testosterone lead to low libido, loss of interest, or even depression.

- The quality of sleep diminishes. Adrenaline is a neurotransmitter that stimulates the brain. If a person is under stress with too much adrenaline, the brain is overactive at bedtime, and it is hard to relax and fall asleep. Poor sleep leads to fatigue, poor memory, and irritability.

- Excessive adrenaline increases muscle contractions, which leads to neck and back pain, as well as tension headaches. Poor sleep further reduces the muscles' ability to rest and relax. Stress has much to do with fibromyalgia, which has two major characteristics: muscle pain all over and insomnia.

- With adrenal fatigue, the immune system also becomes compromised, which leads to more frequent colds and flue. Furthermore, it becomes increasingly difficult to bounce back from illness. Lower immunity also makes individuals more prone to other diseases, including cancer.

At this second stage, a person can still function in high gear, but fatigue starts to set in more often, and many people need to drink coffee or other stimulants to keep going. Weight gain is common, as are diseases such as hypertension, heart attacks, diabetes, fibromyalgia, hypothyroidism, depression and anxiety.

Third Stage Adrenal Fatigue

The third stage of adrenal fatigue is exhaustion. This is the final stage when people become very fatigued and have difficulty functioning at all. At this stage of adrenal exhaustion, life becomes difficult. Blood pressure can become low due to low aldosterone, cortisol and adrenaline; people can feel dizzy especially when changing posture. Recovery from this stage is a long, slow process of equal parts medical treatment and a commitment to lifestyle changes that reduce stressors.

Symptoms of Adrenal Fatigue

Difficulty getting up in the morning.
Continuous fatigue not relieved by sleep.
Craving for salt or salty food.
Increased effort to do everyday tasks.
Decreased sex drive.
Decreased ability to handle stress (anxiety).
Light-headed or dizziness when standing up.
Difficulty recovering from illness or injury.
Depression.
PMS (Premenstrual Syndrome).
Need to drink coffee or caffeinated soft drinks for energy.
Brain fog, not being able to concentrate.
Memory loss.
Irritability.
Inability to sleep through the night.

Frequently, patients with adrenal fatigue are also carrying diagnosis of chronic fatigue syndrome, fibromyalgia, irritable bowel syndrome, hypothyroidism, chronic insomnia, diabetes, leaky gut syndrome, anxiety, or depression.

Diagnosis and Tests for Adrenal Fatigue

It is hard to diagnose adrenal fatigue until its late stage. One reason is the lack of adequate tests. Another is that the symptoms are insidious and overlap with other diseases. But there are several ways to examine the body for this condition:

1. The iris cannot hold contraction when light is shined onto the eye. Normally when we shine a light onto one eye, the iris reacts with contraction of the pupil (making it small) and the pupil remains contracted. In adrenal fatigue, the pupil will not be able to hold its contraction and will dilate despite the light still shining on it. This will take place within two minutes and will last from 30 to 45 seconds before it recovers and contracts again. Sometimes, the iris will contract initially, then dilate, then contract, then dilate again. This inability of the iris to remain contracted occurs in moderate to severe adrenal fatigue, but may not be evident in mild adrenal fatigue. This test is also a good way to determine if an individual has recovered from adrenal fatigue.

2. Low blood pressure and postural hypotension. Adrenaline causes the blood vessels to constrict and raises the blood pressure. Aldosterone causes fluid retention and increased blood volume. It also elevates blood pressure. However, when we develop adrenal fatigue, both of these hormones are low, which results in low blood pressure, unless the blood vessels are rigid and narrowed as a result of atherosclerosis, or hardening of the arteries. When blood pressure is lower than 100 systolic (the high reading) and drops even more when changing from lying down to standing up (postural hypotension), it can cause dizziness, loss of balance and fainting. This condition is very common in adrenal fatigue, and can be aggravated by other conditions such as anemia

or heart failure. With recovery from adrenal fatigue, blood pressure improves and dizziness goes away.

3. Saliva and blood hormone testing. The adrenal hormone levels fluctuate at different times throughout the day. Ideally, levels should be measured four times a day: within one hour of waking, usually from 6 to 8 A.M., when the levels are highest; then between 11 A.M. to 12 noon, again at 4 to 6 P.M., followed by one from 10 P.M. to 12 midnight. Stress levels during the day can affect hormone levels. The blood test measures hormones circulating in the bloodstream. The saliva test reflects tissue hormone levels. We need to check the cortisol and DHEA levels 4 times a day, so the saliva test is used due to its convenience.

Treatment of Adrenal Fatigue

It takes a long time and dedicated effort to recover from adrenal fatigue. In order for the adrenal glands to be restored to optimal levels of functioning, several lifestyle changes are necessary.

Make Sleep a Priority

Sleep is very important for adrenal recovery. For people who have adrenal fatigue, it is best to fall asleep before 10 P.M., because the second wind of adrenal hormone secretion hits around 11 P.M. If you ride on the second wind, which makes you more energetic and prone to stay up until 1 to 2 A.M., you will further exhaust your adrenal glands. Also, not getting up until 8:30 or 9 A.M. helps. This is when the adrenals secrete hormones again; sleeping at this time can be remarkably refreshing.

Steps to help you sleep better:

1. Avoid stimulants such as coffee, tea (except herbal tea), chocolate, or caffeinated soft drinks, especially after noontime. Also, avoid alcohol.

2. Avoid nighttime tension such as fighting with your spouse or children, watching violent movies or television, paying bills, working at the computer, etc.

3. Make your bedroom comfortable without light or noise stimulation. Also make sure it is well ventilated, not too hot or too cold. Make sure the mattress is comfortable.

4. Wear earplugs if your partner snores.

5. Have a sleep routine such as one hour before you sleep, write a daily review or emotional diary. Ask yourself how you feel emotionally. If there is anything that bothers you, write it down, and ask yourself what you can do to handle it. Then ask yourself to release the negative emotions, be it anger or worry. Also write down what you need to do tomorrow and prioritize it. Afterward, do relaxation exercises such as yoga or Pilates, followed by meditation, which slows down the brain waves and leads to sleep.

6. Take supplements like 400-500 mg magnesium citrate at bedtime, which helps relax the muscles for achieving a deeper sleep; and 0.5-1.5 mg melatonin sublingually (under the tongue), which helps to normalize sleep patterns.

7. Other supplements, such as 500-1000 mg tryptophan or 50-100 mg 5-HTP (5-hydroxytryptophan) at night to increase the level of serotonin, which also helps with sleep. Several herbs, such as hops, valerian and licorice, also can help. Hypothalamus extract and adrenal extracts both assist in normalizing sleep patterns.

Take Control of Your Diet—The Adrenal Recovery Diet

1. Reduce high glycemic carbohydrates, which can trigger insulin secretion and leads to hypoglycemia later. This increases the stress load on our adrenal glands. Small, frequent meals help to avoid low blood sugar (hypoglycemia).

2. More salty food is preferable in cases of hypotension (low blood pressure) and dizziness.

3. Breakfast is the most important meal of the day. Plan to eat breakfast every morning.

4. Increase dietary fiber. Using flaxseed meal or psyllium fiber in a smoothie or drink in the morning will help maintain glycemic control, and prevent fatigue in the afternoon.

5. Most people feel fatigued by 4 P.M. when the sugar gets low. Eat a nutritious protein snack with hot herbal tea and sit down to take a few minutes break.

6. Limit caffeine, alcohol, fried foods and sweets.

7. Reduce inflammation by reducing processed and refined food, trans fats and rancid fats.

8. Eat a lot of vegetables with different colors. They are rich in antioxidants, and reduce inflammation. These foods will feed the body with balanced nutrients, including vitamins, minerals, fibers and electrolytes.

9. Eat nuts and seeds as sources of essential fatty acids, which also reduce inflammation.

Reduce Your Stress

1. Simplify your life, set priorities for what you will dedicate your time and precious energy to accomplish. Do not feel guilty if you are not perfect.

2. Journal your moods and emotions each day, and release negative emotions. Also write down what you need to do the next day; being organized will reduce stress.

3. Exercise regularly, particularly relaxation exercises such as yoga or Pilates, which you can do even when you are tired. Stretching exercises help to relax the muscles and reduce muscle spasms and pain.

4. Deep breathing is one of the easiest, yet most effective ways to relax. Combined with the visualization of peaceful settings, deep breathing can do wonders for the body (see pages 209-212 for details).

5. Meditation. Picture a cup filled with water and sand. Shake the cup and the water becomes murky. But let the cup sit for a while and the sand settles down at the bottom of the cup and the water becomes clear again. Meditation helps the mind to become clear. While meditating, let thoughts come through you and do not dwell on any particular thought, just let it pass through. Gradually, the mind will calm itself and thoughts will become less frequent, as the brain waves become slower. You can use meditation before sleep if you have a hard time falling to sleep (see pages 209-210 for details).

6. Find things you enjoy doing and do them regularly. Simple things such as taking a walk along the beach, listening to your favorite music, gardening, dancing, a nice bath or massage, picking flowers, having lunch with a friend, and so on will help you relax and enjoy each day.

7. Do not dwell on the negatives, which have a way of building on themselves and dragging you down. Think positively; appreciate what you have. Gratitude helps keep the focus on the positive aspects of life and assists in responding to life dynamically.

8. Build quiet time into your day. Slow down, take a break, and even lie down after lunch for a refreshing rest.

9. Laughter is the best medicine. Watch comedies, joke with friends, and be silly.

10. Build healthy relationships. Avoid people who are energy robbers.

11. Build financial security. Create a plan. Simplify your life. Get out of high interest debt. Save 10 percent of your income and invest wisely.

Supplements for Recovery from Adrenal Fatigue

Vitamin C

Vitamin C is the most important of all the vitamins and minerals involved in adrenal metabolism, as it is essential to the manufacturing of adrenal hormones. Vitamin C also increases adrenal function and it stimulates the immune function.

The best vitamin C occurs in nature, as this source of vitamin provides the bioflavonoids that enhance its antioxidant effect. Humans do not make vitamin C so it must be derived from food sources, including colored vegetables such as green leafy vegetables and tomatoes, as well as citrus fruits. The highest amount of vitamin C is in the sprouts of any seed and grain. The younger the plant, the more vitamin C it contains.

In the case of adrenal fatigue, vitamin C from food alone may not be sufficient. However, unless you can drink several pounds of fresh juice that you make for yourself daily, it is much simpler to take 500-1,000 mg. of vitamin C with bioflavonoids (at a 2:1 ratio) two to three times a day. Do not stop vitamin C suddenly. Taper it gradually, as you require less as you recover from adrenal fatigue.

Vitamin E

Vitamin E is not directly involved in the metabolism of adrenal hormones, yet it is essential in an indirect way. Manufacturing of adrenal hormones creates harmful free radicals, which slow down the enzyme proteins and damage adrenal glands. Vitamin E absorbs and neutralizes free radicals. It takes both vitamins C and E working together to keep the adrenal glands functioning at optimal levels.

It is important to choose the right type of vitamin E. Most vitamin E sold in stores is d-alpha-tocopherol, but the type of vitamin E needed for adrenal regeneration is beta-tocopherol. Taking mixed tocopherols (d-beta, d-gamma, and d-delta) with vitamin E is important. Take 800 IU a day with meals.

B Vitamins

- **Pantothenic Acid**

  One of the B vitamins, pantothenic acid, is essential for the production of energy. The body converts it into acetyl-CoA, a substance critical for the conversion of sugar (glucose) into energy in the mitochondria inside the cells and tissues. Adrenal cells need a lot of pantothenic acid because much energy is needed for adrenal hormone production. 1,500 mg a day is recommended.

- **Vitamin B6**

  Vitamin B6 is a helpful cofactor in the manufacturing of hormones by the adrenal glands. Take 50-100 mg a day for moderate to severe adrenal fatigue.

- **B Complex**

  The entire B complex is needed in small quantities throughout the production of adrenal hormones. Food sources of B complex are whole grains, miso, brewer's yeast, liver and rice bran. When buying B complex, it is important to buy it in the proper proportion of 50-100 mg of B6, 75-125 mg of B3 and 200-400 μg of B12.

Other Supplements

- **Magnesium**

  Magnesium is also involved in energy production, and adrenal recovery depends on the presence of magnesium.

Vitamin C, pantothenic acid, magnesium, and others work together for adrenal function. Food sources of magnesium include brown rice, nuts, seeds and kelp.

- **Trace Minerals**

Trace minerals include zinc, manganese, selenium, molybdenum, chromium, copper, iodine and some others. They typically have a calming effect and are best taken at night. The best food sources of trace minerals are sprouts, algae and sea vegetables, such as kelp. Liquid minerals are easier to absorb. The best ones are made from natural sources.

- **Fiber**

Fiber helps the body eliminate fat-soluble toxins and thus protects and improves adrenal function. Food sources can be obtained from most vegetables, fruits, seeds and whole grains.

- **Herbs**

There are a few herbs, called adaptogens, which help the adrenal glands to function better. They include licorice root, Siberian ginseng, ashwagandha root, and ginger root. These herbs improve energy and the sense of well-being, but they can raise blood pressure if a person is already hypertensive.

- **Adrenal Cell Extract**

Adrenal cortical extracts are from the adrenal cortex of bovine (cows). The first recorded use of bovine adrenal extract was in 1918, and it has been commercially available since then. Its action is to support and restore normal adrenal function by providing the essential ingredients for adrenal repair. The extract includes adrenal cell contents and nutrients in the form and proportion used by adrenal glands and contains only small amounts of the adrenal hormones themselves. The extract is generally safe and helps to rebuild adrenal glands.

- **IV Nutrition**

  Intravenous nutrition treatments with mega doses of vitamin C, B12, B6, pantothenic acid, B complex, magnesium, calcium, zinc, chromium and selenium are very helpful when people are deficient in those nutrients, and need a quick boost for their energy levels.

Hormone Treatments

- **Testosterone**

  Testosterone implants are very effective in reducing the symptoms of adrenal fatigue. It gives people more energy and mental clarity faster than any other treatment.

- **DHEA and Pregnenolone**

  DHEA and pregnenolone are adrenal hormones. I use them in small doses and monitor blood levels.

- **Cortisol**

  Synthetic cortisol became available in 1950 and has somewhat replaced the use of adrenal cell extract. It is more effective and creates dramatic improvement. However, the down side is that long-term use can suppress our own adrenal function instead of helping adrenal recovery if a high dose is used. For this reason, cortisol should be used only in cases of severe adrenal fatigue and taken only in appropriate physiological doses. Otherwise, side effects may occur and it may become very difficult to safely wean a patient off this product. It is also important to increase the cortisol dosage when the body is more stressed. Never stop cortisol suddenly.

Adrenal fatigue is very common. Most people have mild adrenal fatigue, and are able to recover from this condition with adequate sleep and lifestyle changes. People with moderate to severe cases can still recover, but it will take more work and time.

Points to Remember

1. Adrenal fatigue is very common, especially around mid-life. It is due to long-term physical and/or emotional stress.

2. There are different stages (arousal, adaptation and exhaustion), and different degrees of adrenal fatigue (mild, moderate, and severe).

3. The major symptom of adrenal fatigue is fatigue. Symptoms can range from difficulty getting up in the morning to not being able to function at all. It may also be associated with other diagnoses such as chronic fatigue syndrome, fibromyalgia, hypothyroidism, irritable bowel syndrome, chronic insomnia, diabetes, anxiety or depression.

4. The diagnosis of adrenal fatigue can be challenging. Saliva testing for cortisol four times a day is the current recommended test. Checking blood cortisol to DHEA ratio is another method.

5. The treatment of adrenal fatigue focuses on stress reduction, improving quality of sleep, a healthy diet to reduce inflammation, and the avoidance of blood sugar fluctuation.

6. Moderate to severe adrenal fatigue need supplements to help the adrenal glands produce adrenal hormones. This includes high dose vitamins such as C, B complex and E, also trace minerals such as magnesium, zinc and selenium.

7. Herbs and adrenal cell extract helps to rebuild the adrenal glands.

8. The adrenal hormone, cortisol, is available by prescription, but has to be used with caution and reserved for patients with severe adrenal fatigue. It needs to be used in physiological doses and should never be discontinued suddenly.

CHAPTER 7

Hypothyroidism—The Hidden Epidemic

Anna's story:

My name is Anna, age 57. About ten years ago, I was diagnosed with hypothyroidism (low levels of thyroid hormone) by my family practitioner in North Carolina. She told me I had the thyroid of an 80-year-old and treated me with thyroid replacement hormone. A few months later, I relocated to Florida. My new doctor thought my thyroid was okay and discontinued it. So, I thought my problem had been corrected. Thereafter, my health gradually began to decline, until a few years later I no longer had energy to do the things I enjoyed in my daily life.

I could not maintain my strenuous workout routine, a daily activity alternating between resistance training and cardiovascular exercise. I caught every flu and cold bug circulating in my professional and social environment, and I stayed sick much longer than normal. I was losing so much hair, the vacuum cleaner clogged every time I swept the carpet. I was more sensitive to cold. I gained weight, even though I ate a very healthy, carb-conscious diet. All of these symptoms were compounded by the fact that I also entered menopause, which I thought was the culprit for my decline. I certainly had the typical hot flashes and night sweats that accompany its onset. My quality of life plummeted. Some mornings, as I drove out of my driveway headed toward a very busy day at the office, I cried because I already was so totally exhausted. I simply could not imagine how I would make it through the day.

I went to great lengths to research my health problem, spending thousands of dollars and expending a few years trying to get to the bottom of my difficulties, with no clear-cut results. Then, I heard about bio-identical replacement hormones that were in the form of pellets implanted in the rear hip area. The physician who managed this treatment was one of only three doctors in Florida to do so, but fortunately just minutes from my home. When he reviewed my lab work, he confirmed—at long last—my low thyroid hormone levels were contributing to my health problems.

As an adjunct to pellet implantation, he prescribed 30 mg daily of Armour thyroid and subsequently raised it to 60 mg. Since then, I have lost 30 pounds, my energy levels have returned to normal, I no longer shed hair at prodigious rates, and I am able to maintain the active lifestyle that I prefer. The combination of SottoPelle® pellets and thyroid medication has given me back the quality of life that I so deeply missed during the five years that it took for me to find the reason for my physical decline. No more 80-year-old thyroids in my 57-year-old body, thank goodness!

Hypothyroidism

Our hormones work together. The thyroid, ovaries (women), testicles (men), and adrenal glands are particularly related to each other and have overlapping functions. By the time men and women reach mid-life, it is quite typical for the adrenal and thyroid glands to become very overworked due to the stresses of daily living, environmental toxins, and the aging process. Many people, especially women, are diagnosed with thyroid problems. But, like Anna, even more are just approaching the threshold of diagnosis and spend years suffering without knowing they have mild hypothyroidism, or subclinical hypothyroidism.

Hypothyroidism affects our bodies from head to toe, impacting all of the body's major systems and contributing to chronic diseases. Amazingly, millions of people with hypothyroidism do not show any signs or symptoms and go undiagnosed for years with this problem. According to the American Association of Clinical Endocrinologists (AACE), subclinical (borderline) hypothyroidism—or early stages of decline of the thyroid—is a common disorder, affecting anywhere from 1 to 10 percent of the adult population, with greater impact on women. Furthermore, the AACE says that as much as 20 percent of the population over the age of 60 is affected by this silent condition. That means one in five in this age group is afflicted.

In order to better understand this often undetected health problem, let us first look at how the thyroid works.

Functions of Thyroid Hormones

The thyroid gland is shaped like the letter "H" or, better yet, like a butterfly. The central connection of the left and right lobes, or wings, of the gland and sits just below the Adam's apple (voice box), right up against the windpipe. The two wings fit snugly onto the sides of the windpipe.

Thyroid hormones increase the metabolic activities of almost all the cells in the body in a very complicated way. This gland's elaborate revving up of our cells keeps our bodies humming.

Thyroid hormones increase the number of mitochondria within our cells. Think of the mitochondria as tiny power plants that generate energy for cellular activities. If the mitochondria are deficient due to low levels of thyroid hormone, cells do not receive the energy they need to properly function. That is why fatigue is a major symptom of low thyroid levels.

When children are lacking in thyroid hormones, their development is adversely impacted. These hormones are absolutely essential to prevent the stunting of growth in children, including mental retardation.

Thyroid hormones also affect our digestive system by stimulating carbohydrate and fat metabolism. They increase the absorption of glucose (sugar) from the intestines and break down the glucose to generate energy. In addition, they decrease the body's tendency to store fat by increasing the oxidation (breakdown) of fatty acids. Low thyroid hormones contribute to elevated levels of cholesterol and triglycerides, which can clog the arteries and lead to atherosclerosis. When the thyroid gland is working well, it tends to increase cholesterol excretion in the bile. It is important to know that with thyroid replacement medications, cholesterol and triglyceride levels diminish.

Thyroid hormones impact the gastrointestinal system in other ways, as well. They stimulate peristaltic motion (intestinal muscle rhythm to move fecal matter through the bowels) and the secretion of digestive enzymes. Low thyroid levels lead to constipation and indigestion.

The body's basic metabolic rate is governed by the thyroid. One of the most reliable indicators of hypothyroidism is a low body temperature. A healthy thyroid increases blood vessel blood flow, cardiac output, and increases the number of heart beats per minute. An extremely low thyroid function leads to heart failure.

Brain function also relies on a healthy thyroid system. Low thyroid leads to depression, slow thinking and excessive sleepiness.

Our muscular systems rely on healthy levels of thyroid hormones for increased strength and tone. Low thyroid levels cause muscle weakness.

The normal functioning of the reproductive systems are also impacted by the thyroid gland. Lack of thyroid hormones in women leads to low libido (sex drive), infertility, and irregular menstrual periods. Men will have decreased libido, as well.

Causes of Hypothyroidism

There are several factors that cause the thyroid glands to malfunction, or to slow down their release of thyroid hormones.

First, there are genetic causes. Much like diabetes, thyroid problems tend to run in families, especially in women. If our mothers, grandmothers, or sisters have thyroid problems, it is highly likely that we will have those problems too.

A second cause of hypothyroidism occurs when our immune systems malfunction. The immune system normally produces antibodies to attack foreign invaders, usually proteins from bacteria or viruses. But sometimes our immune systems become confused and produce antibodies that attack our own bodies' cells, targeting different organs. For example, Hashimoto's thyroiditis—also known as chronic lymphocytic thyroiditis—results from these attacks of a person's own immune system on the thyroid gland. This leads to the underperformance of the thyroid gland known as hypothyroidism. Conversely, Graves' disease, which also results from an abnormal immune system attacking the thyroid stimulating function, causes hyperthyroidism or the overproduction of thyroid hormones.

In the case of Hashimoto's thyroiditis, the thyroid hormone initially leaks out of the thyroid gland and elevates thyroid levels. But as the thyroid gland is destroyed over time, hypothyroidism sets in. In most of these individuals, the thyroid hormone levels have not been high enough to cause symptoms of hyperthyroidism. Instead, they are diagnosed with hypothyroidism when the thyroid gland reaches a stage of destruction where it is no longer generating enough hormones.

Iodine is the nutrient our body uses to make thyroid hormones. Iodine deficiency occurs only in areas where the water supply lacks iodine, and should not be common now due to the wide availability of sea salt and seafood. However, it is estimated 25 percent of the women have low iodine levels in their bodies. There are several different causes, such as restricted salt intake in the case of hypertension, drinking distilled water, or exposure to chlorine or fluoride, which can compete with iodine and reduce iodine absorption into the thyroid gland. A deficiency in iodine often leads to goiter.

Another significant factor contributing to hypothyroidism comes from the adverse effects of environmental toxins. There are not sufficient data to know for certain the long-term effects of common chemicals in our environment that infiltrate our bodies. But there are many toxins that have been implicated. These toxins have infiltrated our food and water supplies; namely, pesticides, plastics, and PCBs (polychlorinated biphenyls) that are used as coolants and flame retardants in many household products.[57,58,59] An accumulation of these active synthetic chemicals in our bodies leads to the disruption of the physiologic function of our own hormones, including the thyroid hormones.

Other environmental sources of toxins come from chlorine or bromine added to the water in our hot tubs and swimming pools, and from chlorine, bromine or fluorides added to our drinking water. With the abundance of fluorides in our tap water and in the toothpaste we use every day for the prevention of cavities, our bodies are more likely to accumulate higher levels of these chemicals, which contribute to the slowing of thyroid activity.

A rare condition that can cause hypothyroidism is when the pituitary gland, the master hormone gland located at the base of the brain, underperforms. The pituitary gland secretes thyroid stimulating hormone (TSH) to stimulate thyroid gland to make thyroid hormone. Low levels of TSH cause the thyroid gland to slow down, which then results in hypothyroidism.

Symptoms of Hypothyroidism

Fatigue
Weakness
Slow movements
Weight gain or difficulty losing weight
Sleepiness
Sluggish thinking, poor memory and concentration
Depression and anxiety
Constipation
Cold intolerance, cold hands and feet
Loss of sex drive (libido)
Headache/migraine
Aches and pains in muscles or joints
Irregular periods
Hoarseness

Signs of Hypothyroidism

Low body temperature
High cholesterol levels
Dry skin and brittle nails
Hair loss or thinning of eyebrows
Delayed relaxation of deep tendon reflexes
Infertility
Myxedema (a skin and tissue disorder that leads to puffiness around the eyes, swollen lips, thickening of the nose, non-pitting edema, and yellow skin)

Diseases Frequently Associated with Hypothyroidism

The thyroid gland is central to the healthy functioning of the entire body. When it malfunctions as with hypothyroidism, it can contribute to the onset of other debilitating diseases, such as:

Diabetes mellitus/insulin resistance/obesity
Chronic fatigue syndrome
Fibromyalgia
Allergy or multiple chemical sensitivities

Autoimmune diseases such as celiac disease, lupus or rheumatoid arthritis
Depression
High cholesterol, hypertension and heart diseases
Chronic joint pain and arthritis
Menopause
Infertility

Diagnosis of Hypothyroidism

In my training as an internal medicine specialist, I was taught that there are several tests for hypothyroidism but only need to check the levels of thyroid stimulating hormone (TSH). TSH is secreted by the pituitary gland to regulate thyroid function, and if this regulating hormone is found to be in the normal range, there is no thyroid problem.

This sounds simple enough, but in reality many patients have signs and symptoms of hypothyroidism even when lab results show normal ranges of TSH. This is what occurred with Anna, whose new doctor viewed her as a "hypochondriac" when she insisted that her thyroid was the cause of her health problems.

Years after my residency training, I learned that TSH is not an accurate test for hypothyroidism. Our thyroid gland secretes T4 (thyroxin, which is tyrosine with 4 molecules of iodine). T4 is not an active hormone, so after it enters into the cell one iodine is removed forming T3 (triiodothyronine), which is the active form of the hormone. However, there are many factors affecting the conversion of T4 to T3 and sometimes T4 becomes reverse T3 (the wrong iodine is broken off) instead of normal T3. This explains why the TSH test may be normal—the T4 seems adequate, yet the patient has signs and symptoms of hypothyroidism due to the underlying fact that T3 levels are still low.

Research shows that emotional stress or physical illness blocks the conversion of T4 to T3. Patients with adrenal fatigue usually show normal T4 but reduced T3. Other conditions that can reduce T4 conversion to T3 are unstable blood sugar and insulin levels, autoimmune thyroiditis, and certain drugs.

In my practice, I use several tests to check thyroid function. These tests include TSH, free T3 (triiodothyronine), and free T4 (thyroxine). Thyroid antibodies, such as anti-TPO, are checked for the possibility of auto immune thyroiditis. If indicated, urine iodine is checked after an oral iodine/iodide challenge test to see if there is a possibility of low iodine.

Another very important but simple diagnostic tool involves charting the basal body temperature when a patient has signs and symptoms of hypothyroidism. The patient's body temperature is taken immediately upon awakening before engaging in any physical activity. If it is consistently lower than 98° F, chances are the thyroid function is low.

In addition, if I detect lumpiness or thyroid gland enlargement (goiter) just below the patient's Adam's apple, I obtain an ultrasound scan to check for thyroid nodules or other abnormalities.

Treating Hypothyroidism

1. Medication

The first successful treatment of hypothyroidism was recorded in 1891 in England with the use of desiccated porcine (pig) thyroid gland extract. This was the most effective form of treatment until the 1960s, when pharmaceutical companies began mass production of medications to simulate T4. This treatment has since dominated the medical treatment of hypothyroidism and is prescribed under such brand names as Synthroid, Levoxyl, and Unithyroid.

These medications, however, are not cure-alls for hypothyroidism. The problem is that T4 needs to be converted in the body to T3 to perform thyroid hormonal functions. A pharmaceutical firm subsequently developed Cytomel, a patented T3, to help patients who do not respond well to the T4 medications. But Cytomel is short acting and needs to be taken twice a day.

Interestingly, the original medication, desiccated porcine thyroid, which is now prescribed as Armour thyroid, seems to be quite effective. A study published in 2001 followed 89 patients who were taking T4 medications and then switched to desiccated thyroid.[60] They were followed for two years and their symptoms of hypothyroidism were then compared to their symptoms before the switch. Fatigue dropped from 90 percent to 26 percent; constipation, from 40 percent to 14 percent; depression, from 61 percent to 23 percent; and cold intolerance dropped from 86 percent to 24 percent.

It is fascinating to note that the symptoms of hypothyroidism did not greatly improve with previously administered T4 medications. With desiccated thyroid, however, there was remarkable improvement in all symptom categories. The reason is probably the existence of T3 and other thyroid hormones, T1 and T2, which may well have their own therapeutic functions too.

But remember, everyone is different. Environmental toxins can block the cascade of endocrine and immune actions, making some individuals very sensitive to even small doses of thyroid medication. Other hormones such as sex hormones and adrenal hormones also affect thyroid hormones; people with adrenal fatigue can react adversely to thyroid hormones unless they also receive adrenal hormones at the same time. Or, like in Anna's case, they are treated with female bio-identical hormones and thyroid hormone simultaneously. Anna, who opted to take this route experienced a phenomenal rebound.

Sometimes we may have to try different thyroid medications, if one form does not work well, and increase the dosage gradually until the desired result is achieved. It is also important to take thyroid medication on an empty stomach because foods, especially those high in calcium, reduce the absorption of thyroid hormone.

2. Nutrition

A patient with hypothyroidism may benefit from nutritional supplements, such as selenium, iodine, zinc and magnesium, but thyroid hormone medication is usually the first choice of treatment since thyroid hormones affect digestion. A person suffering from hypothyroidism does not digest or absorb nutrients well.

In addition to thyroid medications, however, a balanced and healthy diet is always recommended. Some foods and substances should be avoided entirely, as they can directly interfere with thyroid function, such as impeding the conversion of T4 to T3. These are caffeine, alcohol, tobacco and sugar.

Specific foods, such as seaweed (kelp) and seafood are important for thyroid hormone production. They contain the trace minerals such as selenium, zinc, iodine and proteins that are needed for the manufacture of thyroid hormones. Replacing table salt with sea salt is another simple way to get iodine.

I recommend the nutritional supplements in the following daily dosages: zinc (20 mg); selenium (200 mcg); and iodine (150 mg). Herbs, such as ashwagandha and Guggul (Commiphora mukul), may improve the conversion of T4 to T3.

3. Detoxification

As mentioned before, thyroid hormones are interrupted by many environmental toxins, such as pesticides, plastics, heavy metals, and water with fluoride and chlorine. Toxin avoidance is the first step, followed by detoxification as discussed in Chapter 11. It is important to improve constipation by using more fiber, magnesium, and the proper dose of thyroid hormones, as fecal excretion is one of the major routes of detoxification and many patients with low thyroid function have constipation problems.

4. Stress Reduction

When stressed, our adrenal glands secret higher levels of cortisol. These higher levels inhibit the conversion of T4 to T3, leading to a reduction in the levels of the active form of the thyroid hormone, T3. For stress reduction, please see pages 267-270.

5. Hormone Balance

All hormones work together. Thyroid hormones are particularly affected by adrenal and sex hormones. Optimize those hormones and you will feel wonderful again.

Self-assessment for Hypothyroidism

Here is a simple test to help you determine if your thyroid gland is functioning optimally.

1. Do you often experience fatigue? Do you wake up feeling tired? Does exercise fatigue you?

2. Do you have cold hands and feet? Do you often need to wear socks to bed?

3. Do you have trouble losing weight, even with little food and lots of exercise?

4. Are you mentally sluggish, forgetful or mentally foggy?

5. Do any of your family members have thyroid problems?

6. Do you suffer from dry skin, brittle nails, or hair loss?

7. Are you experiencing significant menopausal symptoms?

8. Do you have irregular periods or difficulty getting pregnant?

9. Do you have multiple allergies or chemical sensitivities?

10. Do you have chronic constipation and/or indigestion?

11. Do you have bouts of depression or anxiety?

12. Do you have diabetes, hypertension, or high cholesterol?

If you answered "*yes*" to more than four questions, it increases the likelihood that you have borderline or undetected hypothyroidism.

Points to Remember

1. A normal thyroid function test result does not exclude the diagnosis of hypothyroidism.

2. Signs, symptoms, and family history of thyroid problems support a diagnosis.

3. Menopause, adrenal fatigue, and hypothyroidism often occur simultaneously.

4. Many factors can affect the conversion of T4 to T3, the active thyroid hormone.

5. Avoid environmental toxins as much as possible in order to prevent a deleterious effect on the thyroid gland.

6. Avoid fluoridated tap water and toothpaste with fluorides.

7. Avoid exposure to chlorinated or brominated water in swimming pools or hot tubs.

8. T4 treatment alone is often ineffective. Many people need a mix of T3 and T4.

CHAPTER 8

HGH, DHEA, and Melatonin

In recent years there has been a growing amount of media attention and consumer interest in the use of human growth hormone (HGH), DHEA, and melatonin for supplementation. Advertisers have been quick to tout the benefits of these substances, claiming a wide variety of benefits that encompass everything from enhanced sports performance to slowing down the aging process. But what are the real facts behind these so-called miracle supplements and what, if any, benefits can they offer those currently on bio-identical hormone therapy? In this chapter we are going to go beyond the marketing hype and catchy slogans by taking an in-depth look at the scientific facts behind HGH, DHEA, and melatonin.

Human Growth Hormone

HGH is a protein structure made up of 191 amino acids that is secreted by the pituitary gland in the brain. The function of HGH is to promote growth by helping the transportation of amino acids into cells, and the synthesis of amino acids into new cellular structures, especially bones and muscles, as well as internal organs. It is essential in childhood and our young adult years for the purpose of growing bigger and taller. HGH secretion reaches its peak by a person's late teens and declines gradually after that. By the age of 60 or 70, we only have 15 to 20 percent of the hormone levels we had in our peak years.

Since all adults stop growing at some point, it makes sense to ask: Why would we still need HGH in our older years if we are not growing anymore? The answer can be found in HGH's primary function, the synthesis of amino acids. HGH is still needed to help our bodies use the amino acids we ingest to repair cellular damage and generate new cells.

There are quite a few benefits claimed by those who use HGH supplements. Some of these benefits include younger looking skin, stronger bones and immune system, improved muscle mass and cardiac output, increased energy, enhanced sexual performance, sharpened memory, and balanced mood. If some of these benefits sound strangely familiar to you, it is because we have been talking about them in conjunction with pellet therapy all along. As a matter of fact, similar effects can be achieved by implanted bio-identical estrogen and testosterone pellets, which are also hormones that promote growth.

Recent news headlines reported that high-profile athletes in Florida were using HGH illegally in an attempt to improve their sports performance. However, the truth of the matter is that in adults with normal levels of growth hormone, raising levels too high will cause problems like carpel tunnel syndrome, diabetes, or even acromegaly, a medical term for enlargement of bones in the jaw, hands, and feet.

But what about claims that HGH slows down the aging process in men and women? Is growth hormone really the fountain of youth everyone has been searching for? In my opinion, before the age of 60 or 70, hormone replacement with testosterone and/or estradiol pellets will accomplish all this, as they have been proven to improve energy, memory, sexual performance, muscle strength and exercise endurance. After age 70, there may be a role for HGH replacement. It should be cautioned, however, that there are currently no long-term studies on the issue. In addition, if you already have cancer cells existing in your body, HGH will make the tumor or cancer grow faster. For those individuals who do choose HGH therapy, it is important to always use a low dose, monitor hormone levels regularly and have annual physicals, especially cancer screening tests.

Another drawback to HGH replacement is its high cost and inconvenient application. Because HGH has 191 amino acids, making it a fairly large molecule, it is not able to enter our body through the skin or digestive tract. The only way to receive HGH is through daily subcutaneous injections, just like insulin given to patients with diabetes. The cost is also very high, about $500 to $1,000 a month depending on the dosage used.

What most people do not realize is that there are natural ways to increase the amount of HGH our body produces. In fact, by following the advice in this book, you are probably doing it right now. Proper nutrition and daily exercise are the two primary vehicles by which our body can naturally increase HGH production and the amount that it releases. We know that nutrients and amino acids such as arginine, ornithine, tyrosine and methionine contribute to HGH production and release. Strenuous aerobic exercise 30 minutes daily also stimulates the release of growth hormone. By exercising daily and putting wholesome, nutritious foods in your diet you are well on your way to assisting your body in optimal HGH production. For patients who have yet to do this, I recommend starting an exercise program, preferably with a strong aerobic component, and taking amino acid supplements in the morning before exercise.

DHEA

As mentioned in chapter 6, DHEA is an adrenal hormone that can convert into sex hormones. When our cortisol levels are high due to stress, DHEA can help to balance it out. However, the best way to reduce cortisol levels is to reduce stress, or improve our stress coping skills. DHEA can also increase brain function and improve our immunity. It is my opinion that these effects are not just due to DHEA itself, but the conversion of DHEA into sex hormones.

DHEA can be obtained over the counter and, as far as supplements go, is quite inexpensive. Interestingly, it has also been touted as a hormone with anti-aging effects. Yet despite its low cost and the possibility of additional benefits, I personally feel that the anti-aging effect can be achieved much more effectively and safely through implanted testosterone and/or estradiol pellets. This view has been borne out in my practice, where I have observed patients taking over the counter DHEA who achieved negligible results, as well as others who suffered side effects ranging from acne to prostate cancer.

In considering supplementation with either HGH or DHEA, it is important to keep in mind that all hormones are potent and can have consequences well beyond their intended effects.

Do not use hormones by yourself without checking with your physician first. If your physician approves, be sure to monitor your hormone levels closely.

Melatonin

Melatonin has gained popularity in recent years for its use as a sleep aid. Melatonin is a hormone secreted by the pineal gland in the brain. Its prefix, "mela" means dark or black and is so named because our body starts to secret this hormone when it gets dark, helping us to feel relaxed and fall asleep. It also helps us achieve deeper and more restful levels of sleep. The secretion of melatonin declines with age—that is why seniors do not tend to sleep as deeply as younger adults.

Sleep is essential to our health. I usually recommend supplementation with melatonin to patients who are experiencing sleep problems. In addition to being a natural sleep aid, melatonin has other health benefits. Most importantly, it is a free radical scavenger, which means it neutralizes free radicals and reduces free radical damage. Therefore, it helps the body achieve healthy aging through several different pathways.

Melatonin can be obtained over the counter and is inexpensive. Nevertheless, there are still some important rules to observe when supplementing with this hormone. Using the right dosage is especially important. Start with a small dosage, such as 0.5 mg before sleep; gradually increase to 1 or 2 mg, if needed, to achieve better sleep. More than 3 mg is too much and may cause side effects, such as nightmares or drowsiness. Taking too much melatonin also may suppress the body's own production of melatonin.

Melatonin can be taken two ways—sublingually or orally. The sublingual form is preferable, because it bypasses the liver and enters the bloodstream directly. Melatonin taken sublingually lasts approximately 8 hours, and will not cause the hang over effect that sometimes results from taking it orally.

When considering supplementation with HGH, DHEA or melatonin, it is important to keep these facts in mind and remember that our body has natural ways of producing these important hormones. It is also helpful to remember that treatment with bio-identical hormone pellets can provide the same benefits of supplements like HGH and DHEA in a far more effective, safe and sustainable manner. If you do decide to supplement with additional hormones, be sure to check with your doctor first and have your hormone levels monitored closely.

Part III

The Body, Mind, and Spirit Connection

CHAPTER 9

Nutrition—You Are What You Eat

There are all kinds of diets: the Zone diet, Pritikin diet, South Beach diet, Mediterranean diet, Okinawa diet, low-fat diet, low-carb diet, and vegan diet. The list goes on and on. For a long time, it has been considered sinful to eat fat. Now everyone is shying away from carbohydrates and sugar. So, what is left to eat?

Consider the nutrients derived from food. They are carbohydrates, proteins, fats, vitamins, minerals, enzymes, and fibers. All carbohydrates turn into sugar (glucose) as the source of immediate energy for the body. All proteins turn into amino acids, which are the building blocks of cellular structures, hormones and neurotransmitters. Fats turn into fatty acids, which are also building blocks for cellular structures and hormones in the body. Vitamins and minerals are involved in all of the body's chemical reactions, including the detoxification systems. The body secretes enzymes to digest food, and, fortunately, many fruits and vegetables are also loaded with enzymes to help digestion. Fibers help with the elimination of solid wastes. Thus, all of the nutrient groups have their functions, and including each group in our diet is important for our optimal health.

While the basic nutrient groups have remained the same over the millennia, the way humans eat has changed significantly over the past 50 years. As a result of this, problems occur because we have altered our diet from the way that was designed for us genetically over millions of years of evolution. Unlike our primitive ancestors, we eat food that has been processed, refined, bleached, radiated and loaded with food colors and preservatives. We eat food that is even grown differently, due to commercial farming practices that rely on artificial fertilizers, toxic pesticides, and in some cases, genetic modification. This food, unfortunately, generally has a much lower nutritional value than the more natural foods that our ancestors ate. Our food not only gives us poorer nutrients, but is also laced with substances that are toxic to our health. Worse yet, we over eat and our bodies turn this excess of calories into fat.

Breakdown on Nutrients

Let us look more closely at how the nutrient groups in food work in the body.

Carbohydrates

Carbohydrates are made of sugar molecules chained together. There are two types of carbohydrates: simple and complex. Complex carbohydrates are made of three or more sugar molecules chained together, while simple carbohydrates are just one, or two connected sugar molecules. Complex carbohydrates are found in whole grains, vegetables and legumes. Examples of simple carbohydrates are fruits, cookies, cakes and candy. All carbohydrates are broken down in the digestive tract and then absorbed as sugar. Simple carbohydrates, with shorter chains of connection, break down more quickly and are absorbed right away.

Processed carbohydrates come from foods that are refined, such as grains or starchy vegetables. For instance, brown rice is converted to white rice when the outer shell is stripped away. The outer shell contains fiber (the complex carbohydrate), which must be broken down by digestive enzymes before the inside of the rice kernel can be digested. Eating refined white rice, which has been converted to a simple carbohydrate, causes the blood sugar to rise much faster than eating brown rice. However, in the end both the brown rice and white rice produce the same amount of sugar.

Another example of refinement is processing the potato into potato chips. In the body, they both convert to sugar fairly fast, but potato chips have other ingredients, such as salt, hydrogenated oil and preservatives that are not good for the body. Also in the process of refinement, the vitamins and enzymes in the potato are destroyed.

The glycemic index has been developed as a tool to measure how quickly the body converts carbohydrates into sugar. The amount of food ingested also matters. The index, times the amount, comes to the total glycemic load. If you eat a small piece of candy, which has high glycemic index, compared to a bowl of rice, which has lower glycemic index but a higher total amount of carbohydrate, the total glycemic load will be higher in the bowl of rice.

The glycemic index, however, is not the only measure of how fast sugar is absorbed. When we combine foods in a meal, such as fiber or protein or fat, the absorption of sugar will be slowed down due to competition for absorption sites in the small intestine. That is why a balanced meal is important.

The key is to eat mostly complex carbohydrates, not the refined foods that alter complex carbohydrates to less healthful and more quickly absorbed simple carbohydrates. Another key is not to over eat. Too much intake of carbohydrates will only be turned into fat and stored in the body, which leads to weight gain and insulin resistance, as discussed in chapter 16.

Examples of sources of good carbohydrates, both complex and simple, are:

Starchy vegetables: carrots, beets, broccoli, potatoes, yams, corn and peas.

Leafy vegetables: spinach, lettuce, chard and kale.

Grains: barley, brown rice, millet, oats, quinoa, rye and whole grain wheat.

Fruit: apples, bananas, berries, oranges, lemons, watermelons and papaya.

Fats

Many people think that eating fat will make you fat. This is a myth. The fact is the body needs good fats, which become fatty acids that are used to make cellular structures and hormones. The undesirable fat that we gain is usually due to eating excessive simple carbohydrates.

- **Fatty Acids**

Fatty acids are the building blocks of fat. All fatty acids are made of long chains of carbon molecules that have to bind with hydrogen molecules. There are three types of fat: saturated, monounsaturated and polyunsaturated.

— **Saturated fat:** All the carbon atoms are saturated with hydrogen atoms.

Sources of saturated fats are butter, cheese, eggs, coconut oil, and fatty tissue from animal meat.

— **Monounsaturated fat:** One site is missing a hydrogen atom.

Sources of monounsaturated fats are almond oil, avocado oil, olive oil, grapeseed oil and canola oil.

— **Polyunsaturated fat:** More than one site is missing hydrogen atoms.

Sources of polyunsaturated fats are flaxseed oil, sesame seed oil, evening primrose oil, wheat germ oil, corn oil, and fish oil.

All of these fats are naturally occurring and safe to eat. Saturated fat has been denigrated in the past, probably due to the deleterious effect of fats that are often combined with high-glycemic-index carbohydrates in foods, such as in cookies, cakes and ice cream.

Another factor is that toxins tend to deposit in animal fat. When we eat animals, such as cows and pigs, we ingest more toxins from their fat. It is important to use organic saturated fats, especially butter. It is also important to use cold-pressed vegetable oils, as heating in the process of creating the oil changes its structure into trans fats, which increases the risk of coronary heart disease by raising the level of "bad" LDL (low-density lipoprotein) cholesterol and lowering the level of "good" HDL (high-density lipoprotein) cholesterol.

- Essential Fatty Acids

  Among the polyunsaturated fats, there are three essential fatty acids: omega-3 fatty acids, omega-6 fatty acids, and gamma-linolenic acid. The term "essential" means that the body cannot make these fatty acids and we need to get them through our diet. These polyunsaturated fats are essential for our hormone production, particularly the prostaglandins, a group of hormones found in virtually all of the tissues and organs of the body. Prostaglandins act as inflammatory mediators, constrict smooth muscles, and sensitize spinal neurons to pain. Lack of essential fatty acids will lead to more inflammation and aging, in part, because the production of good prostaglandins is slowed. Omega-3 is also the building block for cell membrane structures and nervous system formation.

  Sources of essential fatty acids:

  Omega-3 fatty acids: flaxseed oil, walnut oil, and fish oil from salmon, sardines, tuna, and mackerel.

  Omega-6 fatty acids: canola oil, flaxseed oil, grapeseed oil, corn oil, sunflower seed oil, chicken, eggs, and turkey.

  Gamma-linolenic acid: borage oil, evening primrose oil, and blue green algae.

- **Bad Fat**

There are good fats and bad fats. All naturally occurring fats are good fats. Bad fats are damaged fats, usually as a result of refinement processes used to manufacture them. They include:

1. **Hydrogenated Oil**

   This is manufactured by adding an extra hydrogen atom to vegetable oil, which results in an oil that is a liquid in its natural form but becomes solid at room temperature. Margarines and shortenings are examples of hydrogenated oil.

2. **Trans Fats**

   Polyunsaturated fats are good for the body, but when processed with high heat they become trans fats and bad for the body. When extracted with heat, corn oil, for instance, becomes a trans fat. If it is cold pressed, which means that it is manufactured without the use of heat, then it is good for the body. So, always buy vegetable oils that are cold pressed.

   French fries and fried foods are loaded with trans fats due to cooking the food with high heat. Most of the polyunsaturated oils cannot withstand high heat, so do not cook with flaxseed oil or sesame seed oil. Instead, use them in salad dressing. The best cooking oil is saturated fat, such as butter or coconut oil, because it is more stable with heat. Grapeseed oil can also tolerate higher levels of heat in cooking.

3. **Oxidized, Rancid Oil**

   When oil is exposed to air, oxygen binds with the carbon atoms and the oil becomes oxidized. This changes the color of oil as well as its taste and smell. All oil should be refrigerated after opening. Do not use oil that has been opened and sitting in the cabinet for a long time.

When bad fats get into the body, they replace the natural fat in the cell membrane and make it more rigid. The cell membrane is the gateway to all nutrients and hormones. If the cell membrane malfunctions, such as when it becomes more rigid, the nutrients and hormones the cell needs cannot enter. Bad fat also becomes debris that clogs our cells and blood vessels, which leads to premature aging.

We usually get enough omega-6 fatty acids from foods like chicken, turkey, or eggs. Conversely, we usually do not get enough omega-3 fatty acids from our diet, so supplementation is important.

Protein

All protein turns into amino acids and becomes the building blocks for muscles, bones, organs and tissues. The amino acids are also precursors to neurotransmitters. As such, protein is essential for life. There are 20 amino acids in protein. About 10 are essential amino acids, which means that the body cannot make them, so they have to come from our diet. Good protein usually comes with good fat.

Sources of good protein are:

Eggs. You can eat one to two eggs daily. Do not worry about the impact on cholesterol levels. Ninety percent of cholesterol is made by the liver, not derived from dietary sources of cholesterol.

Meat and poultry. Always buy organic or hormone-free meat and poultry. Do not buy processed meat, such as sausages or ham that come loaded with nitrates and preservatives.

Fish and shellfish. Buy fresh fish instead of canned or smoked varieties. It is preferable to consume wild fish or deep sea fish in order to avoid mercury or artificial colors. Farmed salmon is often fed dyes to color its meat.

Cheese. Most cheese is treated with heat, which can damage its fat, so eat it with moderation. Avoid yellow cheese, as it is colored with dye. Buy organic cheese. People who are allergic to milk cannot eat cheese.

Nuts and seeds. They are excellent sources of good protein and good fat. Nut butters are processed, so be careful about preservatives. Nuts are best eaten raw after soaking for eight hours, which will activate their enzymes for easy digestion. Examples of nuts and seeds are almonds, walnuts, cashews, chestnuts, macadamia nuts, peanuts, hazelnuts, pistachio nuts, pecans, pine nuts, sunflower seeds, sesame seeds, and pumpkin seeds. You can grind nuts and seeds, add olive oil and sea salt to use as a salad dressing or a vegetable dip.

Vitamins

- **Vitamin A**

Vitamin A is important for healthy vision and healthy skin. This vitamin is found in both animals and plants.

Animal sources of vitamin A are beef, liver, and butter.

Plant sources are yellow-colored fruits and vegetables, such as yams, pumpkins, carrots and apricots.

- **Vitamin B**

Vitamin B is composed of eight water-soluble vitamins, including B1 (thiamine), B2 (riboflavin), B3 (niacin), B5 (pantothenic acid), B6 (pyridoxine), B7 (biotin, also called vitamin H), B9 (folic acid) and B12 (cyanocobalamin). The B vitamins are also found in animals and plants. These vitamins are essential for cell functions, especially in the central nervous system. A deficiency of the B vitamins can lead to such diseases as anemia, nerve cell damage, fatigue, PMS (premenstrual syndrome), hormonal imbalance, and malabsorption.

Animal sources of vitamin B are chicken, fish, pork, beef, eggs, and milk.

Plant sources are nuts, seeds, lentils, whole grains, potatoes, leafy green vegetables, corn, mushrooms, broccoli, and beans.

- **Vitamin C**

Vitamin C is important for wound healing and immunity. It helps with the formation of collagen and maintaining youthful skin. Collagen is the main component of fascia, cartilage, ligaments, tendons, bone and teeth. Vitamin C is also a strong antioxidant that neutralizes the free radicals that lead to inflammation. Thus, it slows down the aging process and also plays an important role in the body's detoxification process.

Vitamin C deficiency leads to increased bruising, poor wound healing, and scurvy. Scurvy leads to spongy gums and bleeding from all mucous membranes, as well as the formation of liver spots on the skin. As the disease progresses, individuals lose their teeth and have open, pus-filled wounds.

Sources of vitamin C come from plants only. Humans cannot make vitamin C, and depend on foods such as citrus fruits, cantaloupes, tomatoes, cabbage, and broccoli as a source of this vitamin.

- **Vitamin E**

Vitamin E is an important antioxidant that helps stabilize cell membranes. It protects against lipid peroxidation, which is the breaking down of cell membranes. Vitamins C and E work together to reduce inflammation and to prevent atherosclerosis (hardening of the arteries). There are eight forms of vitamin E. The most common is alpha tocopherol, but delta and gamma tocopherol also have synergistic effects.

Deficiency of vitamin E leads to cellular oxidation and to formation of plaque in the arteries. Vitamin E is important for cardiovascular and brain health.

Animal sources of vitamin E are egg yolks and various fats.

Plant sources are leafy green vegetables, vegetable oils, whole grains, and legumes.

- **Vitamin D**

Vitamin D plays an important role in the absorption of minerals, such as calcium, magnesium and phosphorus. Vitamin D deficiency leads to osteoporosis. Recent studies suggest that vitamin D may protect against autoimmune diseases, such as multiple sclerosis, and different forms of cancer, including breast, colon and prostate.

Low vitamin D is also associated with mood issues such as depression.

Vitamin D is produced by exposure of our skin cells to the sun. Food sources are cod liver oil, liver, and egg yolks. Milk and many cereals are fortified with vitamin D.

Minerals

- **Calcium**

Calcium is important for healthy bones and teeth, but its most important role is in the cell membrane for activating enzymes, neurotransmitters, and hormones. Calcium is also involved with nerve conduction, muscle contraction, blood pressure regulation, and many other metabolic functions. One type of blood pressure medication is called a calcium channel blocker, which blocks the influx of calcium into cells and reduces blood pressure. In cardiac arrest, calcium gluconate is used to stimulate heart contractions.

Because calcium is so important for many life-preserving activities; when it is needed, the body will pull the calcium stored in bones for use in the circulatory system. Thus, insufficient calcium leads to osteoporosis.

Animal sources of calcium are fish or sardines with bones, chicken, milk, cheese, yogurt, and egg yolks.

Plant sources are tofu, beans, broccoli, green vegetables, nuts, and seeds.

- **Magnesium**

Magnesium is also a very important mineral because it involves important metabolic functions, especially energy production in the mitochondria (energy units inside cells). Magnesium relaxes muscles, reduces blood pressure, prevents constipation, and improves mood and sleep. Magnesium deficiency leads to an irregular heartbeat, muscle spasms or pain, irritability, and nervousness.

Magnesium is primarily derived from plants such as beans, broccoli, and avocados, as well as fruits such as lemons, apples, figs, and grapefruits.

In my practice I use magnesium citrate (400-800 mg daily) to treat many conditions such as palpitations, high blood pressure, constipation, muscle cramps, insomnia and anxiety.

- **Chromium**

Chromium is involved in glucose metabolism and has been shown to improve insulin sensitivity (increases the body's response to insulin so less is required). This makes it a very important supplement for people who have diabetes or sugar craving.

Animal sources are meats, eggs, and cheese.

Plant sources are nuts, mushrooms, beets, and legumes.

- **Selenium**

Selenium works with vitamin E and helps in stabilizing the cell membrane. It is also an antioxidant involved in liver detoxification. Studies show selenium helps prevent cancer, diabetes, and heart diseases. It also boosts one's immunity.

Selenium deficiency is often due to heavy metals that can inactivate this mineral. Heavy metals that interfere with its function include cadmium as a result of smoking or exposure to batteries, mercury from eating certain fish or as a result of dental amalgam fillings, and/or lead due to exposure to industrial and automobile pollution.

Animal sources of selenium are tuna, salmon, meats, and other seafood.

Plant sources are fresh garlic, wheat germ, whole grains, and mushrooms.

- **Zinc**

Zinc is another essential antioxidant mineral that is involved in many cellular functions and enzyme pathways. Studies show that zinc helps to protect the eyes from blindness due to macular degeneration, improves arthritic conditions, and enhances immune function.

Animal sources are chicken, pork, turkey, beef, liver, eggs, seafood, and milk.

Plant sources are wheat germ and pumpkin seeds.

- **Iodine**

Iodine is very important in the production and regulation of thyroid hormones. Low levels of iodine lead to hypothyroidism and goiter (enlarged thyroid gland). Iodine is also involved in many enzyme systems involving energy production, nerve function, breast health, hair, and skin growth.

The best food source is seaweed, especially kelp, sea salt, seafood, and iodized salt.

- **Potassium**

Potassium plays a major role in maintaining tiny electrical currents in the cells, especially heart and muscle contractions, and nerve transmission. Low potassium levels lead to an irregular heartbeat, muscle cramps, weakness, and even mental confusion. Rapid IV (intravenous) infusion of potassium will cause the heart to stop.

The best food sources for potassium are fruits like bananas and oranges. Other plant sources are apricots, lettuce, broccoli, potatoes, nuts, seeds, wheat germ, and other fresh fruits.

Animal sources are liver and fish.

- **Iron**

Iron is essential for the formation of hemoglobin, which carries oxygen from the lungs via red blood cells to the body. Iron is also found in myoglobulin, a molecule in the muscles that transports oxygen to muscle tissue. A lack of iron leads to anemia, which is more common in women before menopause.

Animal sources of iron are liver, meats, and shellfish.

Plant sources are leafy green vegetables, whole grains, fruits, and nuts.

Fiber

Fiber is the structural material of plants that performs a function similar to the skeletal structure of animals. It is important for the GI (gastrointestinal) tract, as it is the food source of friendly bacteria in the large intestine. There are two types of fiber: water-soluble and water-insoluble.

- **Water-soluble Fiber**

  Water-soluble fiber plays several important roles:

  — Slows down the entry of carbohydrates into the blood stream, thus it reduces blood sugar and insulin secretion. That is why eating water-soluble fiber is very important for individuals with diabetes or insulin resistance.

  — Helps detoxification by binding heavy metals and other toxins.

  — Helps to lower cholesterol by binding the cholesterol in the bile and food.

  Sources of water-soluble fibers are vegetables, fruits such as apple, and carrots. The mucilage of legumes and seeds also contain water-soluble fibers.

- **Water-insoluble Fiber**

  Water-insoluble fiber has very little effect on sugar absorption or insulin secretion. It does increase the bulk of stool, which helps with elimination, detoxification, and preventing constipation.

Fiber is found in all plant sources such as fruits and vegetables, whole grains, nuts, seeds and legumes.

Enzymes

The body secretes enzymes to digest food. Many fruits and vegetables contain enzymes that help with digestion. Cooking food at a temperature of over 118° F, however, will destroy the enzymes provided in food. In fact, cooking food at a temperature above 160° F will destroy all vitamins in the food. This is why we should attempt to eat the majority of our fruits and vegetables raw.

Water

Up to 70 percent of the body is made of water, which really is our number one nutrient. There are two types of water in the body: intracellular water and extracellular water.

- **Intracellular Water**

  Intracellular water is water within the cell and is needed for all cellular functions. More water is maintained in the cells (over 60 percent of the total) the younger we are. As we age, we maintain less intracellular water. That is why children's skin looks like freshly picked grapes, while seniors look like raisins. Less intracellular water leads to reduced cellular function and lowered metabolism. The cell membrane determines whether or not water can get into the cell. A soft membrane is more water permeable, while a rigid one is not.

  To improve intracellular water, we need to improve cell membrane permeability by eating foods with more essential fatty acids, as they are the building blocks of cell membranes. Another factor is toxins in the body, because more toxins in the tissue draw water out of the cell. Removing toxins by detoxifying the body will help the permeability of the cell membrane.

- **Extracellular Water**

  Extracellular water is the water that circulates in the bloodstream and between cells. Too much extracellular water leads to water retention and edema. Not enough water in the circulatory system causes dehydration, which has serious consequences such as fatigue, weakness, light-headedness, and fainting.

Water quality is also a problem. It is not a good idea to drink tap water, as chlorine and fluoride are added to the water supply. Other chemicals, such as fertilizers, pesticides, as well as organic chemicals such as PCBs and benzene can leak into the water supply from the environment. The quality of drinking water can be controlled by installing a home water filtration system.

Whatever you health goal is, you can customize your diet to fit your needs. The principle of a healthy diet is one that gives us adequate nutrition and also reduces inflammation.

Anti-inflammation Diet

There are 6 key concepts to reduce inflammation:

1. Reduce sugar load. High glycemic index carbohydrates increase insulin secretion. Insulin triggers inflammation reactions.

   — Avoid refined carbohydrate foods and foods with a high glycemic index.

   — Eat small meals about every 3 to 4 hours.

2. Reduce toxins in the food.

   — Avoid processed foods, which have artificial food colors, sweeteners, preservatives, and MSG.

   — Eat organic foods to avoid pesticides, herbicides, and xenohormones.

3. Increase omega-3 fatty acids from salmon, avocados, nuts or seeds to reduce inflammation. Avoid trans fats, hydrogenated oil and rancid oil from foods such as hamburger, french fries, cookies, and brownies, which cause inflammation of blood vessels.

4. Increase anti-oxidants from fruits and vegetables of all colors. Anti-oxidants neutralize free radicals and reduce inflammation.

5. Increase fiber and water to assist the body's detoxification processes.

6. Use herbs such as ginger, garlic, rosemary, and turmeric, which have an anti-inflammation effect.

Weight Loss Diet

This diet is focused on reducing insulin and reducing inflammation.

1. Reduce your total calorie intake. Check your metabolic rate. Most people will be able to lose weight with a diet of 1,000 to 1,400 calorics a day.

2. Our body prefers to use sugar as our energy source. If you keep on eating carbohydrates, you are not going to burn fat. It is a good idea to eat mostly protein initially to switch our body's energy utilization system.

3. Drink lots of filtered water (about 50 percent of your body weight in ounces).

4. Avoid high glycemic index carbohydrates, especially from refined white flour products such as pastas, cakes, cookies, pretzels, donuts, white bread, white rice, pizza, noodles, etc. Avoid foods loaded with sugar, including candies, baked goods, fruit juices, soft drinks, ice cream, etc. These foods stimulate insulin secretion and the more you eat the hungrier you get. This is a big "NO NO" if you want to lose weight and improve metabolic syndrome.

5. Avoid bad fats from processed foods (potato chips, popcorn, etc.), fried foods (french fries, fried chicken, etc.), processed meats (bacon, sausages, hot dogs, ham, smoked or cured meats, etc.), rancid oil, trans fats, and saturated fats.

6. Eat the fresh organic vegetables listed below as much as you like. Eat them mostly raw. Vegetables provide abundant enzymes, antioxidants, minerals and fiber. Cooking destroys enzymes and vitamins.

Green leafy and cruciferous vegetables, including alfalfa sprouts, bok choy, broccoli, cabbage, cauliflower, chard, collard greens, kale, lettuce, and spinach.

Other vegetables are asparagus, bean sprouts, bamboo shoots, bell peppers, celery, cucumbers, green beans, mushrooms, onions, peas, radishes, string beans, sprouts, summer and winter squash, tomatoes, zucchini, and sea vegetables (kelp).

7. Eat good protein and good fat, such as organic nuts, seeds, avocados, chicken, turkey, and wild salmon. Remember the serving size, not more than 3 ounces, and the methods of cooking include baking, broiling, and grilling.

8. You can have whole grains (oatmeal, brown rice, millet, etc.), fruits (apple, berries, oranges, grapes, pineapples, etc.), and legumes (garbanzo beans, kidney beans, black beans, lentils, etc.), but eat only one group at each meal and be careful about your portions. These foods are healthy, but they still contain quite a bit of carbohydrates.

9. Condiments: Cinnamon improves insulin sensitivity, so use it generously. Turmeric, ginger and garlic have anti-inflammation effects, so use them frequently too.

Healthy Aging Diet

1. Reduce inflammation, as discussed above.

2. Do not over eat. A famous study done in 1935 showed the life span of laboratory rats could be extended by 50 percent with serious calorie restriction. While in humans this can be unrealistic, the goal of avoiding over eating is achievable.

3. Choose your fat wisely. Essential fatty acids, especially omega-3 fatty acids, are used to make hormones and cellular structures. Increasing good fats, such as fatty fish, supplements of fish oil, flaxseed oil, along with nuts and seeds, helps to increase hormone production, improves immunity, and reduces inflammation.

4. Increase growth hormone production by increasing the intake of amino acids, such as protein shakes, especially before exercise.

5. Optimize digestion and absorption by eating raw fruits and vegetables that come with enzymes. Eat fermented food such as yogurt or sauerkraut for the healthy bacteria that protect the intestinal tract. Have vinegar with salad to increase the stomach acidity. Eat mindfully and chew well.

Points to Remember

1. Eat balanced meals, as all nutrients have important functions.

2. Eat smaller meals, snack in between meals if you are hungry.

3. Never over eat, but do eat when you are hungry.

4. Reduce inflammation by avoiding high intake of sugars and fatty foods.

5. Eat foods in their natural forms and try to avoid processed or refined foods. Eliminate artificial food colors, sweeteners, and preservatives.

6. Eat fresh organic fruits and vegetables of all colors.

7. Cooking destroys enzymes and vitamins; eat raw vegetables and sprouted foods for their increased nutritional value and supply of enzymes.

8. Eat fresh organic nuts and seeds as sources of proteins and beneficial fats.

9. Eat unprocessed organic meat, eggs, chicken, butter, and wild salmon. Eat meats and seafood no more than three times a week.

10. Eat fermented foods, such as yogurt, soy yogurt, sauerkraut, and miso soup to promote friendly bacteria in the intestinal tract.

11. Avoid trans fats, hydrogenated oils, and rancid oils. Avoid cooking with vegetable oils and use butter or coconut oil instead. Avoid all deep fried foods.

12. Buy cold-pressed vegetable oils.

13. Avoid high-glycemic-index carbohydrates, especially processed foods made of white flours and sugar.

14. Make an effort to increase intake of essential fatty acids.

15. Drink plenty of filtered water. Aim to drink 50 percent of your body weight in ounces each day.

16. Fibers help the body to detoxify, as well as reduce cholesterol, slow down the absorption of sugar, and lower the release of insulin. All fruits, vegetables, and whole grains provide fiber.

17. Add herbs such as garlic, ginger, cinnamon, and turmeric for seasoning because of their high nutritional value and anti-inflammation effect.

Take the time to evaluate your current diet to find out for yourself whether the foods you are eating are helping you to live longer and healthier, or if they are hindering you from reaching your full potential for well-being. By taking the steps needed to evaluate and improve your diet, you will not only help your body to resist disease and age slower, you will be making invaluable progress toward your goal of living each day with optimal clarity, energy, and zest.

CHAPTER 10

Intestinal Health—Our First Line of Defense

The GI Tract

Good nutrition depends not just on what we eat, but also on how healthy the GI (gastrointestinal) tract is. If the GI tract does not work well, it does not digest food or absorb nutrients very well. Like the skin that protects us from the outside world, the GI tract is the first line of defense against harmful bacteria, viruses, fungus, or toxins in the food we ingest.

Components of the GI Tract

The GI tract is a major system of the body and consists of:

- **Mouth and Teeth**

  The functions of the mouth and teeth are receiving food, chewing to break the food down into smaller particles and mixing these particles with saliva, which secretes enzymes to split complex carbohydrates (starches). It is important to chew food thoroughly and to keep your teeth and gums healthy. A poor state of oral health where loose and lost teeth are common will adversely affect your ability to chew thoroughly. Infection in the gums can cause low-grade inflammation and even heart valve infection.

- **Esophagus**

  The main function of the esophagus is to swallow so that chewed food will move from the mouth down to the stomach. The epiglottis is an elastic cartilage tissue that sits over the vocal cords. It closes during swallowing to prevent food from going down the windpipe and causing choking. This is a very serious risk for the elderly because choking can cause aspiration pneumonia, which results from accidentally inhaling food or liquids. Avoid talking or laughing when your mouth is full.

- **Stomach**

The stomach further mixes chewed and salivated food into chime, and digests protein by secreting HCl (hydrochloric acid) as well as the enzyme pepsin. The stomach only digests proteins, not carbohydrates or fats. Eating sugar without protein will not utilize the HCl, thus causing the stomach to remain acidic and often leading to acid reflux back up into the lower esophagus, which creates heartburn. When digestion in the stomach is not functioning properly, we experience symptoms such as heartburn, bloating, and belching. In addition, insufficient stomach digestion also leads to problems with flatulence and discomfort in the large bowel. Over-the-counter antacids and medicines, such as Zantac or Prilosec, are most commonly used to treat bloating, gas, dyspepsia (heartburn), and acid reflux. Use of these medicines can be greatly reduced by avoiding simple sugar, eating more protein, and taking digestive enzymes as well as hydrochloric acid.

- **Pancreas**

The pancreas manufactures and releases digestive enzymes. Pancreatic enzymes are released via the pancreatic duct into the duodenum (first part of the small intestine beyond the stomach) for the digestion of foods. The enzymes trypsin and chymotrypsin digest protein into amino acids; amylase digests starch into sugar; and lipase digests fat into fatty acids. Insulin is also secreted by the pancreas to handle the sugar load in food and to help transport the sugar from the bloodstream into the cells.

- **Liver**

The liver is the chemical factory of the body. After all the foods we eat are digested and absorbed, the nutrients go directly to the liver, where sugar is converted into glycogen to be stored as a future energy source. The liver also converts the glycogen back into sugar for use when the body requires it. The liver stores vitamins such as vitamin A, D, E, K, and B12. It manufactures bile to store in the gallbladder. The liver is also the body's major detoxification center. It converts fat-soluble toxins into water-soluble forms, so the toxins can be carried through the bloodstream to the kidneys for excretion in the urine or through the bile duct to the intestines to be eliminated as stool (feces).

- **Gallbladder**

This is the storage place for bile, which emulsifies fat. People who have their gallbladders taken out may have problems digesting fat and may develop bloating and diarrhea.

- **Small Intestine**

The small intestine has three sections: the duodenum, jejunum and ileum. The final breakdown of fats, proteins and carbohydrates takes place in the duodenum. Ninety percent of the absorption of nutrients occurs in the jejunum and ileum. Problems in this area will lead to malabsorption and malnutrition.

- **Large Intestine**

The horseshoe-shaped large intestine consists of the ascending colon, transverse colon, and the descending colon. The major function of the large intestine is absorbing water, short chain fatty acids, and vitamins produced by beneficial bacteria in the colon. The large intestine also eliminates feces.

Beneficial Bacteria

At birth, the GI tract is sterile. Shortly thereafter, bacteria start to colonize the large intestine. These friendly bacteria are symbiotic with the body. Their total number exceeds that of our own cells. They feed on the fiber we eat and produce fatty acids and vitamins, particularly the B complex vitamins, for use by our bodies. They form a slimy layer on the intestine wall, where they help to prevent the overgrowth of yeast, viruses, and toxic bacteria.

The protection provided by healthy bacteria is very important. As we age, beneficial bacteria decrease in number. They are also destroyed by frequently taking antibiotics, having frequent intestinal infections or food poisoning. At such times, it is important to reintroduce friendly bacteria by eating fermented foods such as sauerkraut, yogurt, or soy yogurt. Taking probiotics (healthy bacteria such as acidophilus) also helps.

We need to eat 25-35 grams of fiber each day to feed friendly bacteria. Since the body produces a lesser amount of enzymes and absorbs fewer nutrients with aging, it is also a good idea to take digestive enzymes to aid with the digestion of food.

Leaky Gut and Food Allergies

This is a group of disorders not usually emphasized in medical textbooks. Most doctors are not very aware of this disease category. Yet, patients with this problem suffer tremendously. They go from doctor to doctor without getting the right diagnosis or treatment. The more problems they have, the more medications that are prescribed for them, and pretty soon they become walking pharmacies. Unfortunately, this predicament only tends to make the sick become sicker.

How do people get this type of disease? It starts either from a dysfunctional gut or from excessive exposure to toxins, and in many instances the combination of both.

We absorb nutrients through two pathways: diffusion and active transport. Diffusion is a simple process. Substances of different concentration equilibrate and reach the same concentration. Electrolytes, such as sodium, potassium, magnesium, bicarbonate, and chloride get into the body in this way. But most nutrients such as amino acids, fatty acids, glucose, minerals, and vitamins enter the body through active transport, which means the body produces carrier molecules that actively carry the nutrients into the intestinal cells.

The linings are very tight between the cells so that large molecules or unwanted substances cannot make their way into the body. Think of this as a secured gate of a house, which only opens for guests but not for uninvited people. When uninvited people enter the house, the alarm will be activated and a fight will begin to take place. When unwanted foreign molecules or large food particles get into the body, the body produces antibodies to fight those molecules. This process causes inflammation, which wrecks more havoc on the body.

Leaky gut is a disease syndrome caused by an impaired intestinal defense system that allows toxins, large undigested food molecules, unwanted chemicals and microbes to get into the body. This then triggers all kinds of diseases and symptoms, ranging from allergies, acne, asthma, autism, eczema, irritable bowel syndrome, ulcerative colitis, autoimmune diseases, arthritis, headaches, fibromyalgia, mood swings, foggy mind, memory loss, multiple chemical sensitivities, and premature aging.

There are several ways that the body's intestinal defense system is impaired or destroyed, which can then cause a leaky gut.

1. Antibiotics

The first antibiotic, penicillin, was discovered in 1928 by Scottish scientist Sir Arthur Fleming and later developed for use as a medicine by Australian Nobel Laureate Howard Walter Florey. Penicillin saved the lives of many people who would have otherwise died from infectious diseases. After that, numerous antibiotics were manufactured. Now they are given liberally whenever we have a cold, flu, bronchitis, sinusitis or urinary tract infection. These antibiotics kill both good and bad bacteria, so that long-term or frequent use of antibiotics destroys the protective healthy intestinal bacteria and opens the door to the overgrowth of resistant bacteria, parasites, viruses, and fungi such as candida. These unhealthy microbes often form chemicals that are poisons in the body, such as ammonia, hydrogen sulfide, indoles, and phenols that not only damage the intestinal mucosa lining but also enter into the bloodstream, causing a large variety of diseases and symptoms.

Candida is a fungus found in our environment and in the body. It is normally kept under control by friendly bacteria, the immune system and the intestinal pH. When candida anchor and colonize the intestinal mucosa, they secrete toxins that enter into the bloodstream directly. These toxins contribute to inflammation, bloating, fatigue, headache, mental fog, and other symptoms. They also damage the intestinal cell lining so that large undigested food molecules can enter the bloodstream, which triggers the formation of antibodies. While these antibodies are working to fight the food molecules, they can also damage our own tissues, and cause autoimmune diseases.

2. Pain Medications

NSAIDs (non-steroidal anti-inflammatory drugs) such as aspirin, Advil®, Motrin®, Aleve® and ibuprofen are the most commonly sold over-the-counter (OTC) medications. Prescription medications such as Naprosen, indomethacin, Voltaren, Toradol, and Celebrex® are also in this group. The latter are more potent than the OTC pain medications.

NSAIDs work by blocking prostaglandins, which are a group of hormones involved in the body's process of healing and repair. Certain prostaglandins can also increase inflammation and pain. Accordingly, there are good and bad prostaglandins. NSAIDs indiscriminately block all of them. They reduce pain by blocking the prostaglandins that increase pain and inflammation, but they also block the prostaglandins that improve healing and repair, including the intestinal linings, where the cells turn over every three to five days. Thus, one of the well-known side effects of NSAIDs is GI irritation, ulcers, and bleeding. Long-term use of NSAIDs interferes with the healing and repair of the intestinal lining and opens the gate to unfriendly invaders.

3. Poor Eating Habits and Lifestyle

Our diet has a tremendous impact on our GI system:

- A low-fiber diet makes us prone to constipation. As a result, toxins reside longer in the intestines and irritate the intestinal mucosa.

- Processed foods loaded with sugars, hydrogenated oil, trans fatty acids, food colors, artificial sweeteners and preservatives promotc inflammation of the intestinal lining.

- Alcohol and the use of multiple drugs affect the liver's detoxification function and contribute to the accumulation of more toxins in the body, which damages cells in the intestinal lining.

- A stressful and sedentary lifestyle reduces the immune defense system and flow of blood to the intestines. In the long run, every cell in the body is affected and does not function optimally. This includes the intestinal lining cells, especially since they are regenerated every three to five days.

4. Environmental Toxins

The body can only handle so many toxins. If we are continually bombarded with environmental chemicals and heavy metals our bodies will eventually be overwhelmed with toxins. These toxins interfere with cellular functions, including those of the intestinal lining. When the intestinal defense system is lowered, more toxins enter the body. It becomes a vicious cycle.

5. Other Medications and Treatments

Steroids such as prednisone or cortisone are used frequently to treat allergies and autoimmune diseases. Long-term use of these medications suppresses the immune system and increases fungus growth in the GI tract and other parts of the body.

Radiation to the abdominal area as a cancer treatment can damage the intestinal mucosa and cause leaky gut. Most chemotherapy drugs damage the body's cells in general, including the GI tract. This leads to such side effects as nausea, vomiting, and malabsorption.

Diagnosis of Leaky Gut Syndrome

Determining the presence of leaky-gut syndrome involves a combination of the following tests.

1. Intestine Permeability Testing

Lactulose/mannitol test. Both mannitol and lactulose are complex sugar molecules that the body cannot utilize or metabolize. Once ingested and absorbed, they are excreted in the urine unchanged. Mannitol is much smaller than lactulose. A healthy intestine absorbs mannitol easily, but not so with lactulose. Patients with leaky gut absorb a much higher ratio of lactulose compared to healthy people. The test is done by drinking a mannitol and lactulose solution. The urine is collected for six hours and then sent to the laboratory. A high ratio of lactulose/ mannitol indicates the permeability of the intestine is too high, which is consistent with a leaky gut.

2. Comprehensive Digestive Stool Analysis (CDSA)

This test measures the bacterial balance of the intestinal tract and digestive functions. It checks the types of bacteria that are present and measures the levels of beneficial and harmful bacteria. It also checks for the presence of candida and what therapeutic agent is most effective. This test also checks the butyric acid and short-chain fatty acids that are produced by friendly bacteria in the intestines. A low level of short-chain fatty acids means an insufficient amount of probiotics (friendly bacteria). Checking for parasites can also be done with the CDSA, but the result can be unreliable if just done on one random sample. Multiple testing will increase the reliability of the accuracy of the results.

3. Food Allergy Testing

Allergists usually do skin testing or blood testing for IgE antibody-mediated allergies, such as hay fever or asthma. But most food allergies are not IgE antibody-mediated. Checking IgG antibodies is more reliable for food allergies. Other antibodies, such as the antiglidin antibody for wheat allergy and the antibody for candida can be checked with food allergy panels, which can include up to 150 different foods.

Treatment of Leaky Gut Syndrome

The diagnostic tests can be expensive and may not be covered by insurance companies, so a course of treatment can be tried first to see if there is improvement clinically.

1. Assist Digestion of Food

Chew your food well and take digestive enzymes with each meal. This is the easiest and least expensive method of treatment. Digestion starts in the mouth. As we chew, digestive enzymes from saliva are mixing with the food. If you chew the food into smaller particles, it makes the work of the stomach and small intestines much more efficient. Taking digestive enzymes with each meal further aids with digestion and reduces large food molecules as they move into the intestinal walls.

2. Avoid Common Food Allergens

Avoid common food allergens. Eighty percent of food allergies are due to milk, wheat, processed foods, and citrus fruits. You can simply do an elimination diet, by eating only rice, all fruits except citrus fruits, all vegetables except nightshade vegetables (tomatoes, eggplant, potatoes, and red/green/yellow/ chili peppers), fresh herbs (garlic, ginger, oregano, parsley, dill, rosemary, thyme, turmeric), fish, and olive oil. Drink only filtered or mineral water or herbal tea. Eliminate alcohol, soft drinks, coffee, decaffeinated coffee, chocolate, red meats, soy and soy products (tofu, soy milk, soybeans), milk and milk products (ice cream, cheese, cottage cheese, butter, yogurt, cream, and baked food with milk), wheat and wheat products (bread, pasta, cereal, and crackers), all processed foods, artificial sweeteners and condiments. Once you feel better, start introducing one type of food at a time, such as chicken, red meat, nuts, seeds or soy products. Introduce one new food and eat it two to three times a day. If you are feeling fine after a few days, introduce another type. If your old symptoms return, you are probably allergic to this type of food. Once you find the food you are allergic to, avoid it for at least six months and reintroduce afterward. If you get sick again, you may have to permanently eliminate this type of food, which will most likely be milk or wheat products. Finding the foods you are allergic to in this way is very cost-effective. It does take time, patience and persistence to do it correctly.

3. Treat Dysbiosis

Dysbiosis is due to the imbalance of intestinal bacteria flora. There are three types of bacteria: the helpful, the neutral, and the harmful. When there are more harmful bacteria than helpful bacteria, your health is jeopardized. Treatment depends on the type of pathogens you have. Your physician should be able to prescribe the appropriate medication after stool testing. Natural treatments that are effective to eliminate pathogens are garlic, grapefruit seed extract, and oil of oregano in capsules. Candida also responds to natural treatment. A prescription antifungal medication sometimes kills the candida too quickly and large amounts of endotoxins are released into the bloodstream. This will worsen a patient's symptoms. It is a good idea to use a small dosage to begin and gradually increase the dosage as needed.

4. Reintroduce Friendly Bacteria

Dr. Eli Metchnikoff was a scientist who was awarded the Nobel Prize in 1908 for discovering the friendly bacteria called lactobacilli, which can displace many disease-producing bacteria and reduce the toxins they generate. Lactobacilli (found mostly in the small intestines) and bifidobacteria (found mostly in the large intestines) are the two most well studied friendly bacteria.

Humans and friendly bacteria are symbiotic; we supply them with a warm environment and lots of foods (fibers), and in return they produce vitamins that include B1, B2, B3, B5, B6, B12, and folic acids. They also produce lactic acid, which facilitates the absorption of minerals such as calcium, iron, and magnesium. The lactic acid and hydrogen peroxide that these friendly bacteria produce inhibit other harmful microbes. Take probiotics supplements that contain lactobacilli and bifidobacteria, one to two capsules two to three times a day. Most of them need to be refrigerated to keep the bacteria alive. Eating yogurt or soy yogurt helps, but you need a much higher count of friendly bacteria if you have dysbiosis.

Japanese researchers have studied fructooligosaccharides (FOS) and found those sugar molecules can rapidly increase the growth of lactobacilli and bifidobacteria. Many foods have FOS, especially bananas, barley, garlic, onions, asparagus, tomatoes, artichokes, and wheat. Taking probiotics together with foods high in FOS will double the effect.

5. Reduce Toxins

Reduce exposure to toxic substances and use antioxidants to help the body detoxify. Please see Chapter 11 for greater detail.

6. Healthy Diet

See Chapter 9 for more information on nutrition.

Self-assessment for Leaky Gut

Use this questionnaire to gauge your current state of intestinal health.

Answer each question based on the following symptoms:

Point scale:

0 = not present
1 = mild and happen sometimes
2 = moderate and happen often
3 = severe and happen all the time

Section A

______ 1. Do you have constipation and/or diarrhea?
______ 2. Do you have abdominal pain or bloating?
______ 3. Do you have indigestion or reflux?
______ 4. Do you have burping and belching?
______ 5. Do you have flatulence and passing gas?
______ 6. Do you have nausea or vomiting?

[ ] Total Score for Section A

Section B

______ 1. Do you have stomach discomfort when consuming certain foods?
______ 2. Do you have blood or mucous in your stool?
______ 3. Do you pass foul smelling gas or stool?
______ 4. Do you suffer from chronic constipation?
______ 5. Do you experience frequent diarrhea after traveling to another country?
______ 6. Do you have joint pain or swelling?
______ 7. Do you have low energy or become easily fatigued?
______ 8. Do you have hay fever or sinus congestion?
______ 9. Do you have asthma attacks?
______ 10. Do you have ulcerative colitis, Crohn's disease, or celiac disease?
______ 11. Do you have eczema, skin rash or hives?
______ 12. Do you have fibromyalgia or chronic fatigue syndrome?
______ 13. Do you experience mood swings, irritability, mental fog, or memory loss?
______ 14. Do you use antibiotics frequently for urinary tract infection, sinus and respiratory tract infections?
______ 15. Do you use NSAID medications, such as aspirin, Motrin®, Advil®, or Aleve®?
______ 16. Have you engaged in the prolonged use of steroids such as prednisone?

[ ] Total Score for Section B

Interpreting the Results

Section A

If you scored 4 or more in section A, you will benefit from an intestinal health and repair program. The symptoms are due to suboptimal digestion and inflammation of the GI tract. Taking digestive enzymes, probiotics, and fiber with a diet that reduces inflammation may help. If not, seek professional help.

Section B

If you scored 4 or more in section B, you may have intestinal dysbiosis (toxin producing bacteria or yeast in your intestine), food allergies, or leaky gut. You may start the treatment yourself with the plans discussed above. You may also need to seek professional help.

Summary

As we have been able to see, achieving a nutritious, balanced diet is critically important for our everyday health and our body's ability to resist disease. When it comes to our diet, however, eating well is only part of the picture. In order to reap the full benefits of a healthy diet it is equally important to maintain a healthy GI tract. If you have already begun to experience many of the symptoms associated with leaky gut syndrome, then it is of critical importance to restore your intestinal lining back to health, otherwise your current condition many continue to worsen. Just as it makes sense to improve your health through wholesome, nutritious foods, so too will taking care of your GI tract pay enormous long-term dividends on your path to optimum well-being.

CHAPTER 11

Our Toxic World—The Silent Killer

Bio-identical hormone pellets have helped people to experience remarkable improvements in their quality of life by revitalizing the body, balancing the emotions, and clearing the mind. Sometimes, however, addressing hormonal issues alone is not enough to bring patients back to a state of optimal health. As a physician who encourages patients to look at and consider the entire picture when it comes to their health, I know that our bodies can be susceptible to both internal factors and the environment around us. Each day I see more and more patients who reflect this sensitivity, a powerful reminder that our environment has become increasingly toxic and poses continued risks to our health. Take Mary for instance, and the journey towards healing that she undertook when her body began to suffer from the toxic effects of mercury poisoning.

Mary's story:

My name is Mary, and at age 50, my body suddenly "hit the wall." I had previously been extremely active and had been working hard to build and maintain my health as I approached middle-age. I was dedicated to exercising regularly and eating highly nutritious meals. But then I was stricken with a flu that took weeks instead of days from which to recover. I had a lingering cough that just would not go away. My internal medicine doctor diagnosed asthma and prescribed powerful medications that he said I would need to take the rest of my life. After a few weeks, with the irritating cough still persisting, I saw a pulmonary specialist, who told me that I had an asthmatic bronchitis that accompanied the flu virus and was way overmedicated. Nonetheless, he suggested I continue to take the asthma medicine, just at a lower dosage. I did not want to be on that medication at all. Thoroughly disgusted with what I had experienced with these two doctors, I then sought the help of a doctor of Chinese medicine who was able to gradually wean me off of the asthma medicine.

Months later, however, after weekly treatments of acupuncture and cupping, she admitted that she could not understand why that nagging cough would not go away. Every time a cold or flu afflicted someone I knew, I caught it and became terribly sick with a severe respiratory infection followed by the lingering cough. After a year of this suffering, I found a naturopath who diagnosed that my real problem was not in my lungs but, rather, it was due to the many dental amalgams in my teeth. He said that my sudden decline in health, persistent cough and respiratory infections, fatigue (which was not relieved by sleep), depression, and hopelessness was due to mercury toxicity. By now my life had become a matter of doing the bare minimum to get by each day. My naturopath referred me to the team of a biological dentist and physician who specialize in mercury detoxification. Having already spent two years and thousands of dollars trying to find the cause of my decline in health, I was now to embark on a very expensive and horrifying healing journey that entailed as my dentist said, "The replacement of a lifetime of bad dental work in just a month."

Immediately after one or two of the mercury-laced dental amalgams were removed from my teeth, I would go to the physician for IV chelation. This was necessary because, even though my dentist took extraordinary precautions to protect himself, his assistant, and me from exposure to mercury while removing the amalgams, he said that it was impossible for him to prevent incidental exposures. The IV chelation would help my body recover from this toxic exposure. In fact, while my dentist was working on my fillings, a lady visited his office to ask his advice. Having heard of the dangers of mercury toxicity, she had her amalgams removed all at once by a dentist who did not follow the safety protocols practiced by this dentist and physician. She was extremely sick (my dentist said, "her blood was thicker") and she hoped that my dentist would be able to help her. With the damage already done, he told her it was unfortunately too late, she would now have to live with it. In my own case, after the completion of the dental work to replace the silver/mercury amalgams with materials that were biologically friendly to my body, my physician told me it would take a year for me to regain my health.

It was a tough year with several setbacks of painful respiratory infections, but it turned out that my doctor was right. Gradually, my energy returned. I was able to get a good night's sleep and wake up in the morning more refreshed. My immune system began to ward off circulating colds and flu. My life returned to normal. A couple of years later, I encountered a man stricken with mercury poisoning who was confined to a wheelchair. Once a powerful executive, he was unable to talk or walk due to the neurological damage caused by this noxious heavy metal. It was quite scary to think that I could have ended up in that predicament had I not aggressively sought the underlying cause for my lung ailments. I am so grateful that I have had the opportunity to properly and safely eliminate the source of my mercury exposure.

Have you ever wondered why there is such an increased rate of breast cancer and prostate cancer compared to 50 years ago? Or why so many people suffer from allergies?

Have you ever thought about why diseases such as chronic fatigue syndrome, fibromyalgia, or multiple chemical sensitivities were not even mentioned in medical literature 50 years ago? Or wondered about why so many children are diagnosed with autism or attention deficit hyperactivity disorder (ADHD) when in the past these were rare diseases?

Have you ever wondered why there are so many neuro-degenerative diseases such as Parkinson's, Alzheimer's, and multiple sclerosis?

The last century has borne witness to rapid changes in our level of technology, industry and manufacturing processes, more so than in any other century before. Our use of land for agriculture and development, combined with our high demand for fossil fuels has led to a number of significant changes in the environment, including deforestation and ozone depletion. This in turn has had a profound effect on the air we breathe, water we drink, and land we use to produce our food. All of these changes have a direct impact on our health. Consider the following questions:

- Did you know that the average human sperm count has dropped by more than half, from 125 million/ml in 1932 to 50 million/ml in 1998?

- Did you know that there has been a 30 to 40 percent increase in undescended testes and deformed penises in boys over the past 30 to 40 years?

- Did you know that data from the Environmental Protection Agency (EPA) shows that 1.2 billion pounds of chemicals that are potentially harmful to humans were released into the air and water in 1998 alone, and that about 4 billion pounds of pesticides are now used annually in the U.S.?

- Did you know that, since World War II, between 75,000 and 80,000 new synthetic chemicals have been released into the environment? Did you know that on average, more than 400 synthetic chemicals can be found in your body at any given time?

We human beings are conducting a massive, dangerous experiment to see what the chemicals we have invented will do to our bodies, our environment, and our planet. It is not just one or two chemicals, but hundreds and thousands of them combined together.

Rachel Carson wrote *Silent Spring* in 1962. Carson warned in her visionary book that, unless we change what we are doing, there will also be a silent summer, fall and winter. She described how the proliferation and persistence of chemicals were contaminating our environment. Carson also documented how those chemicals accumulated in our bodies. Human beings livinv in such remote areas as Canada's Baffin Island now contaminated with synthetic chemicals such as PCBs, DDT, and dioxin. Since that time, efforts have been made to clean up the environment, but there has not been enough accomplished to alleviate the damage that has accrued over time, nor is enough being done today to prevent further damage.

Three decades after Carson's warnings about the damages accruing from polluting our environment, Theo Colborn, Dianne Dumanoski, and John Peterson Myers wrote *Our Stolen Future* (1996). This book provides scientific research about a wide range of man-made chemicals that disrupt our delicate hormone and metabolic systems. These systems play critical roles in our health, and their disruption can lead to low sperm count, infertility, neurological disorders, and hormone-triggered cancers such as breast and prostate cancer.

Faced with this array of evidence documenting the decline of our environment, we need to ask the important questions: Are we threatening our fertility and survival? If so, what should we be doing about it?

Types of Toxins

With the arrival of the Industrial Age, humankind has managed to compound all manner of chemicals, while helpful to the manufacturing of myriad products, also taint the environment and hence our bodies. These include pesticides, industrial compounds, fertilizers, and heavy metals, among others. Let us take a closer look at some of the major toxins in our environment.

Pesticides

There are three major types of pesticides that have been commonly used over the last century. Many are still in use today.

1. Organochlorides

This is a group of chemicals and pesticides known as chlorinated phenols. The most well-known one is DDT (dichlorodiphenyltrichloroethane), which was first synthesized in 1874. However, its use as a pesticide did not begin until the 1940s, when it was sprayed to control mosquitoes and protect crops. Chlordane was used in pest control for millions of homes from the 1940s to the late 1980s. Heptachlor replaced chlordane, until it was banned in 1978. Even though these pesticides have been banned, they can persist in our environment for decades. Meanwhile, other pesticides in this group are still being used, such as 2, 4-D and 2, 4, 5-Trichlorophenoxyacetic acid. These numerically named organochlorides are commonly used in agriculture and on lawns.

— PCP (pentachlorophenol) is used as an outdoor wood preservative for the treatment of utility poles and railroad ties.

— PCBs and PBBs (polychlorinated biphenols and polybrominated biphenols) were widely used in electrical equipment and transformers in the past and are still used in construction.

— Chloroform (trichloromethane), discovered in 1831, was originally used as an anesthetic drug, but was banned from use in consumer products in 1976. Yet chlorine in the water combined with organic material such as dead leaves produces chloroform. It is found in water treatment facilities and in tap water in many cities.

— Carbon tetrachloride can be found in cleaning products, degreasing agents, dry cleaning solutions, and paints. In the 1940s, it was used in refrigerants and fire extinguishers, but such use has since declined. Its use in consumer products was banned in 1970.

This group of chemicals can cause DNA changes and cancers. These chemicals also damage the liver, kidneys, immune system, and central nervous systems.[61]

Even though it has been banned since 1972, DDT can still be found in human breast milk, blood, urine and sperm. It is also found in many forms of wildlife in many different parts of the planet. In birds, it caused such thin and brittle eggshells that seriously threatened the survival of several species, including the peregrine falcon.

2. Organophosphates

The common group of pesticides, marketed as Dursban, diazinon, parathion, and malathion was designed as a nerve gas to damage the nervous system and kill insects. It can also damage the central nervous system of humans and affect the behavior of both humans and animals, causing symptoms such as blurred vision, confusion, discoordination, and even death. [61,62] The use of organophosphates has also been linked to brain cancer, leukemia, and non-Hodgkin's lymphoma. Dursban has been used widely over the past 20 years for termite control. It was only partially banned in 2001. This group of pesticides has been spayed liberally over different cities for mosquito control, and farmers have used it to control insects. It is still in use today.

3. Carbamates

These are similar to organophosphates but cause less permanent damage. They are being used as fungicides and herbicides. They are also used in clothing, medicines, and plastics. Symptoms such as blurred vision, weakness, memory loss, convulsions, and behavioral problems can occur for several hours after exposure. Other problems, such as thyroid function disturbance have also been reported.

Industrial Compounds and Chemical By-products

Pesticides are not the only toxic chemicals to have infiltrated our environment. Man-made industrial compounds and their chemical by-products have also made a great impact on the world around us. What follows are a few of the major compounds that have achieved widespread integration into our day-to-day world.

1. Phthalates and Plasticizers

Phthalates and plasticizers are found in industrial chemicals such as inks, adhesives, vinyl floor tiles, paints, and plastics such as plastic food wraps, plastic bottles, Styrofoam cups, plastic baby bottles, and plastic food containers. Phthalate from these plastic compounds can enter foods through direct contact, particularly during microwave heating, or when using plastic to wrap hot food.

Bottled water in plastic containers can also be contaminated by these compounds when stored in a heated environment, such as a garage or car. Do not heat frozen foods with plastic containers in the microwave. Do not drink bottled water if it has been sitting in a heated environment for a long time. Do not drink coffee or hot tea in Styrofoam cups. Do not use plastic containers for foods that have been heated. Avoid buying foods in plastic containers such as fruit juices, ketchup, milk, or beverages.

We are exposed to plasticizers every day. They are so thoroughly integrated with the packaging of our foods and our environment that they filter through our bodies day in and day out. These chemicals interrupt our hormone systems, especially the thyroid and sex hormones. They may cause boys to be more feminine.[63] They may also cause precocious puberty (early onset of puberty) in girls. Their long-term effects have yet to be seen, but I truly believe this is one of the major reasons for the increased cancer rate in the reproductive systems, such as breast and prostate cancers.

2. Solvents

Solvents such as benzene, toluene, and xylene are commonly used as cleaning agents and a precursor to the manufacture of dyes, drugs, synthetic rubbers, and plastic products. These solvents are frequently labeled as “inert” and are not listed as ingredients in products, even though they may cause cancer and other serious diseases.

Benzene is a universal solvent used in engine fuels and in the plastics, paint, and textile industries. It may damage bone marrow and thus lead to leukemia. Toluene is used to dissolve many common products, especially ink. Xylene is used in spray paints, plastics, photography, and in the leather and rubber industries. Both toluene and xylene can damage the nervous system, liver, kidneys, eyes, and skin.

Heavy Metals

Heavy metals in our environment can also pose a threat to our health. Heavy metals are not biodegradable and hence accumulate in the environment. They enter the body through our air, water, and food. Once inside our bodies they accumulate in our fatty tissues, central nervous system, and bones. Heavy metals in general inactivate our enzyme systems, increase the production of free radicals, and damage mitochondria in the cells and tissues of the organs. They cause diseases so slowly that it is hard to recognize their impact or to even diagnose until late in the disease process.

1. Mercury

— There is no safe level of mercury for humans. It is among the most toxic substances on the planet, right behind radioactive substances.

— Most people are exposed to mercury through dental amalgam, so-called "silver" fillings, which are composed of 50 percent mercury. Mercury vapors are continuously released from amalgam fillings, especially when eating heated food.

— Most fish are contaminated with mercury due to the polluted waters of their environment. According to the EPA, fish containing the highest levels of mercury are tuna, swordfish, mackerel, shark, halibut, ahi, snapper, and lobster. Fish with medium levels of mercury include sea bass, crab, and flounder. Fish with low levels of mercury are salmon, scallops, and shrimp.

— Other sources of mercury come from additives in cosmetics, thimerosal (preservatives used in vaccines), latex paints, floor waxes, wood preservatives, and various batteries.

Mercury is the most dangerous of all heavy metals. It interferes with mitochondrial function and thus with energy production.[64] Mercury increases oxidative stress and inflammation, as well as damages blood vessel walls and the immune system.[65] It interferes with the liver detoxification pathways. It is a silent killer that cause diseases years after accumulated exposure. The symptoms of mercury toxicity are very nonspecific and, much like those exemplified by Mary's story, may just be fatigue or low immunity. To make matters more complicated, specific tests are needed to reveal mercury in the body—it cannot be found from regular blood tests.

The dangers of mercury in the body are well known to the medical community. Clinically, mercury toxicity has been linked to many diseases that affect crucial body systems:

— **The Central Nervous System**

This is the principle target organ.[66] Some of the diseases of the central nervous system that have been associated with mercury toxicity include:

Autism
Parkinson's disease
Tremor
Dementia and memory loss
Depression
Mental confusion or foggy mind
Neuropathy (numbness, tingling or weakness of extremities)

— **The Cardiovascular System**

Mercury toxicity can adversely affect the functioning of the cardiovascular system. This is due to free radical damage to the vascular system, which causes atherosclerosis.[67] The diseases associated with mercury toxicity are:

Hypertension
Cardiovascular diseases
Myocardial infarction (heart attack)
Stroke

— **Autoimmune Disease or Lowered Immunity**

Our immune systems, which is critical to keeping us healthy and protecting us from diseases, can also be vulnerable to mercury toxicity, leading to conditions such as:

Allergies
Multiple sclerosis (MS)
Frequent episodes of cold or flu

— **Other Diseases**

Mercury toxicity has also been linked to diseases such as:

Chronic fatigue syndrome
Fibromyalgia
Multiple chemical sensitivities
Irritable bowel disease
Cancer

Diagnosis for Mercury Poisoning

There are several ways to determine if your body is suffering from mercury poisoning.

1. History: If you have had multiple dental cavities with amalgam fillings for many years, or if you eat fish more than 3 times a week, you probably have too much mercury in your body.

2. Hair analysis: Testing strands of hair for heavy metals is an easy but not always accurate way to determine mercury levels, as hair only represents recent exposure.

3. Blood levels: If you have high or on-going exposure to mercury then your blood mercury levels will be elevated.

4. RBC (red blood cells) mineral and heavy metals: This is a test that shows mercury in the tissue, but again it is limited to recent exposure as a RBC has only a 90 day life span. Watching mineral levels—especially zinc, selenium, and magnesium—is important because IV chelating may reduce them. When this occurs, these minerals must be replaced.

5. Urine heavy metals: The most accurate test is the urine provocative test. This involves using DMSA (2,3-dimercaptosuccinic acid) or DMPS (2,3-dimercapto-1-propanesulfonic acid) orally or intravenously and collecting the urine for 6 to 24 hours afterwards. This test not only detects mercury, but a

number of other heavy metals such as lead, cadmium, and arsenic. DMSA or DMPS are called chelators due to the fact that they act like a claw, grabbing mercury and other metals as they bring them from the liver through our detoxification systems, where they are eventually excreted in the urine and stool. It is a diagnostic as well as a therapeutic treatment.

Treatment for Mercury Poisoning

If your doctor has determined that you suffer from high levels of mercury exposure, then there a number of ways to help detoxify your system.

1. Remove the source of exposure. If you have amalgam fillings, you need to have them removed. It is always wise to take precautions if you decide to remove dental amalgams because you will be exposed to more mercury vapors in the process. The process for amalgam removal should only be done by dentists who are aware of the best way to prevent additional exposure to this toxic metal.

   Sometimes it is wise to remove only a few amalgam fillings at a time rather than many of them all at once, since the fewer that are removed the less the likelihood of heavy exposure to mercury. In order to help reduce exposure of the body to mercury during the amalgam removal process, IV chelation before and after the removal of silver fillings should also be planned.

   If you have been eating fish or seafood known to have high mercury contamination, you need to reduce the amount you eat and replace them with fish that have less mercury exposure.

2. Chelation with DMPS, orally or intravenously. This is the most effective treatment method, but the draw back is that chelators grab other minerals and metals too, including the ones we want to keep, such as zinc, magnesium and

selenium. It is important to assess and replace these minerals before and during chelation treatments.

It is a good idea to do a Detoxification Capacity Panel blood test to see if your body has the ability to detoxify. It is also important to check for any deficiencies in minerals and fatty acids—be sure to replenish them before beginning treatment. Without careful attention during this process, moving these nasty heavy metals can make you sicker. If you have irritable bowel or leaky gut syndrome, then chelating the mercury through an IV route is better than through oral administration.

2. Lead

Like mercury, lead is a naturally occurring heavy metal that is recognized as an environmental health risk throughout the world. Although the ill-effects of lead toxicity have been recognized for thousands of years, it is still a ubiquitous metal that is used in everything from mining and refining to electrical wiring, paints, and ceramics. Some of the negative effects that lead poisoning can have on the body include:

— Anemia. Lead kills red blood cells by blocking their metabolism, which causes anemia.

— Lead impairs development of the nervous system, which leads to learning disabilities, attention span deficits, and other behavioral problems in children.

— Lead interferes with detoxification enzymes, causing oxidative stress, and cell death.

— Houses built before 1978 can have lead paint and lead plumbing. Other sources of lead exposure include toys, ceramics with lead in the glaze, costume jewelry, leaded gasoline, fishing weights, bullets, and so on.

— After lead is absorbed in the body, it is deposited in the bones. When calcium leaks out of the bone at the time of a fracture or due to osteoporosis, lead seeps out as well. Acute lead poisoning is rare now but chronic, low-level exposure still exists for children and adults. The tests used to detect mercury poisoning can also detect lead and other heavy metals. Hair analysis, blood and urine samples are all useful, especially following a DMSA or EDTA provocation test. Lead can be chelated out of the body much more easily than mercury. Sometimes the use of supplements consisting of 2,000 mg of vitamin C, 50 mg of B6, and 1,500 mg of calcium can eliminate lead from body tissues. IV chelation with EDTA and DMPS are approved treatments for lead poisoning.

3. Aluminum

Aluminum is found in antacids, antiperspirants, pots and pans, aluminum foil, and baking powder. Aluminum is a biochemical that can attach to the phosphates in our DNA.[68] Once it binds with our DNA, the body cannot chelate it out by IV treatments. Excretion is mostly through the feces. There is no proven method for detoxifying aluminum, so avoidance is the best strategy. Avoid aluminum-containing antiperspirants, antacids, aluminum canned foods, and cookware made of aluminum. Keep aluminum foil out of direct contact with food.

Sources of Chemicals In the Environment

The environment we live in today has changed quite a bit from the environment our parents and grandparents lived in. Today, toxic chemicals abound in our food, air and water supply. What follows is a brief listing of some of the most prevalent places such toxins can be found.

1. Foods

Pesticides in our fruits and vegetables.
Hormones in animal meat, eggs, milk, and cheese.

Mercury in fish and other seafood.
Plasticizers in plastic food wraps, bottles, and containers.
Aluminum in aluminum food wraps.
Processed foods contain preservatives, sweeteners, MSG, and artificial food colors.

2. Water

Our water is home to a number of unhealthy chemicals, including fluoride, chloride, plasticizers, and chemical contaminants.

3. Air

Chemicals contaminants can come from sources such as perfumes, car exhaust, gasoline and diesel fumes, sprayed pesticides, cleaning solutions, and paint.

4. Medical and Dental Treatments

Certain treatments, such as vaccinations with thimerosal (ethyl mercury) and dental amalgam mercury fillings are toxic to the human body.

5. Skin Contact

Our skin can also absorb toxic contaminants through everyday household items, including:

Laundry detergents
Cosmetics
Shampoos and hair dyes
Cleaning solutions

6. Environment

Our environment contains a large number of pollutants and chemicals toxins that exist in our homes and items we encounter each day, such as:

Lawn chemicals
Building materials
Carpet
Paints
Wood preservatives
Leather treated with chemicals
Clothing, especially dry cleaned garments
Playgrounds and school yards sprayed with pesticides
Flea soaps or pest collars for pets

Toxin Avoidance—How to Avoid Exposure to Toxins

The following tips will help you take positive steps towards detoxifying your diet and household environment:

— Always buy organic fruits, vegetables, and meat.

— Eat foods in their natural form, not processed.

— Stop eating fish and other seafood that contain high levels of mercury.

— Remove mercury-based amalgam dental fillings.

— Drink water filtered by a process of reverse osmosis or purified by a carbon filter.

— Do not heat foods in plastic containers in microwave ovens.

— Do not use plastic food wrap.

— Use HEPA air filters or ionizers to reduce dust, molds and other indoor pollution.

— Avoid using chemicals to clean your house. Use soap, baking soda, or vinegar instead.

— Do not use pesticides in your lawn, garden, or house.

— Use natural products for shampoos, cleaning solutions, hair dyes, and cosmetics.

— Avoid products that contain aluminum, such as antiperspirants, antacids, as well as pots and pans.

— Keep plenty of house plants to help filter indoor air.

— Do not dry clean your clothes routinely. Be sure to air out dry cleaned clothes before wearing them.

— If you smell anything putrid or acrid, try to clean the source of the smell right away. If this is not possible, try to put a comfortable distance between yourself and the source of the air pollution.

How the Body Detoxifies

Have you ever wondered about the nuts and bolts of detoxification? Just how does our body handle all of the environmental toxins that surround us and assault our internal systems each and every day? The answer involves a bit of biology, but it is actually quite interesting and easy to understand if we focus on the five main pathways of elimination in the body—the liver, kidneys, lymphatic system, colon, and sweat.

Detoxification is the process of the body's biochemical actions to eliminate unwanted chemicals. This process is mainly governed by the liver, which packages the unwanted chemicals to make them less toxic. The packaged chemicals then travel from the liver into the bile and are discharged into the intestines to be removed as feces.

Another route of excreting packaged chemicals is by traveling through the blood stream to the kidneys. Heavy metals and toxic chemicals are then excreted in the urine. Some toxins, especially heavy metals, migrate out of the body through the hair and nails. Another exit pathway for toxins is through perspiration and sweat.

The detoxification system helps the body eliminate extra hormones, neurotransmitters, and a wide variety of toxic chemicals such as drugs, heavy metals, pesticides and plastics. If the body does not detoxify well or is exposed to too many toxins, the toxic chemicals will deposit in the body's tissues and organs, especially in the central nervous and immune systems. These then form the underlying, or root cause of many diseases in the body.

1. The Liver Pathway of Elimination

Detoxification starts at the liver, which is the most important detoxification organ in the body. There are two phases of detoxification in the liver.

— **Phase I**

Phase I involves many protein enzymes, called cytochrome P450 enzymes. The chemical reaction involved is hydroxylation. Phase I produces many free radicals that can harm the body. It is like a waste treatment plant where more toxic intermediate products are produced. The nutrients used at Phase I are:

Riboflavin (vitamin A)
Niacin (vitamin B3)
Pyridoxine (vitamin B6)
Folic acid
Vitamin B12
Glutathione
Branch-chained amino acids
Flavonoids
Phospholipids

— **Phase II**

Phase II detoxification involves conjugation reactions, usually methylation and glucuronization. The Phase II detoxification pathway becomes very important to remove the more toxic intermediate products from Phase I. Lots of antioxidants are needed to reduce the free radicals produced from the Phase I detoxification pathway.

Antioxidants to reduce free radicals at this stage are:

Vitamin A
Vitamin C
Vitamin E
Selenium
Copper
Zinc
Manganese
Coenzyme Q10 (Co-Q10)
Bioflavonoids
Milk thistle
Pycnogenol
Thiols (found in garlic, onions, and cruciferous vegetables such as broccoli and cauliflower)

Nutrients involved in the Phase II pathway are similar to the ones in Phase I, but additionally this phase requires a large amount of amino acids, such as:

Glycine
Taurine
Glutamine
N-acetylcysteine
Cysteine
Methionine

If we want to help the liver to detoxify, it is imperative to take the vitamins, minerals, and amino acids involved in the Phase I and II pathways.

Many enzymes are involved in the liver detoxification pathway, and these enzymes are related to our genetic makeup. For instance many Asians, including myself, are alcohol intolerant. On one occasion, I drank a Mai Tai thinking that it was a non-alcoholic tropical drink. Within half an hour, my face began to flush; I had palpitations and felt very dizzy. These symptoms occurred because I do not have a powerful form of the enzyme acetaldehyde dehydrogenase. After the intestinal absorption of alcohol, it goes straight to the liver where the detoxification process starts. An enzyme called alcohol dehydrogenase converts the alcohol into acetaldehyde, which is 30 times stronger than alcohol. Then the enzyme acetaldehyde dehydrogenase converts the acetaldehyde into acetate (which is converted into fat), carbon dioxide, and water by another enzyme. Many Asians have a genetic variation that results in the production of a less powerful acetaldehyde dehydrogenase. The result is that the effect of alcohol is 30 times stronger for us, since more acetaldehyde stays in our system.

While we are on the subject of detoxification, let us take a look at how our body detoxifies estrogen. Starting in the liver, a Phase I detox pathway involves hydroxylation (OH). The OH can be linked to the number 2, or 4, or 16 carbon. The 2-OH metabolite becomes a weak estrogen, while the 4-OH and 16-OH metabolites still have a persistent estrogenic effect. This is important, because women who metabolize a larger proportion of their estrogen via the C-2 hydroxylation pathway tend to have a lower breast cancer rate compared to women who metabolize through the C-16 pathway. Which enzymatic route a woman metabolizes through is due to her own genetic variation. However, a diet high in cruciferous vegetables (i.e., broccoli, cabbage, and Brussels sprouts) can increase the C-2 hydroxylation pathway, which could reduce the risk of breast cancer.

After hydroxylation, the estrogen metabolites are oxidized to quinones, which become much more toxic to our body. This is the time when the Phase II detox pathway starts. The Phase II pathway involves methylation and glucuronization of the estrogen. The resulting metabolites are then excreted through the feces and urine. Methylation requires B6, B12, folate, and magnesium, so a lack of these nutrients would slow down the detoxification of estrogen. Additionally, the presence of harmful intestinal bacteria can further complicate successful detoxification. Many of the most harmful bacteria have an enzyme called beta-glucuronidase, which can uncouple the glucuronized estrogen and result in the estrogen being sent back to the liver to be detoxified again. Taking probiotics, such as acidophilus, will inhibit the harmful bacteria.

As a result of genetic variations leading to differences in detoxification enzymes, certain people can handle more toxic loads, while others become ill. If you do not have a good genetic make up and do not have enough antioxidants and amino acids to help the enzymes in the detoxification pathways, you will begin to develop health problems if your toxic load is too high. Even a healthy individual with good genes and adequate nutrients runs the risk of developing diseases if their exposure to toxic chemicals is prolonged enough.

2. The Kidney Pathway of Elimination

Our kidneys each contain about one million glomeruli, which are small balls of tiny blood vessels called capillaries. The capillary walls have many extremely tiny holes, which allow particles smaller than the holes to be filtered out of the capillaries into the urinary tract system, while keeping larger particles from escaping. The most common particles that are filtered out are actually water molecules, and more than 90 percent must be reabsorbed back into the capillaries to avoid dehydration. Toxins are filtered out this way, they are not reabsorbed.

To facilitate the excretion of toxins it is important to drink a lot of water. It is recommended that you drink 50 percent of your body weight in ounces. For example, if you weigh 150 pounds, then you should drink 75 ounces of water daily. One glass of water is about eight ounces.

3. The Lymphatic System Pathway of Elimination

The lymphatic system is made of lymph nodes, ducts, tissues, and capillaries connected throughout the body. It is not as structured as the circulation system, which is an enclosed system that has a central pump (the heart). Rather, movement in the lymph system occurs with the milking action of the skeletal muscles when they move (contract), especially near the joints.

Toxins in the body's tissues can be transported to the lymphatic system by exercise or massage, and then excreted as sweat. The lymphatic system can also move the toxins into the circulatory system, where they are excreted in the urine. Exercise helps the body to detoxify by increasing blood circulation and lymphatic drainage. Massage also helps with lymphatic drainage.

4. The Colon Pathway of Elimination

The colon is the body's disposal system. It serves as a temporary holding tank for what the stomach and small intestine did not digest. It is also the normal residing place for more than 400 different kinds of bacteria. The most well known bacteria are Lactobacillus acidophilus and Bifidobacteria, so-called friendly bacteria or probiotics.

Unfortunately, some unfriendly bacteria and yeast also live in the GI (gastrointestinal) tract. Both of these organisms produce many toxins. In such situations, dysbiosis (abnormal bowel germ population) occurs. The harmful yeast or bacteria must be removed or reduced, and probiotics need to be reintroduced to accomplish this.

We should have bowel movements once or twice a day. Constipation slows down the transit time of stool, allowing some of the toxins to be reabsorbed into the body. Chronic constipation means the body is not able to detoxify efficiently.

To assist with moving digested food and eliminated toxins through the intestines, we need 20 to 30 grams of fiber daily. Fiber is the food source of healthy intestinal bacteria. It also prevents constipation, which keeps the toxins from accumulating in the bowels and getting reabsorbed into the body.

— **Good sources of fibers are:**

Flax seed. You can grind these small seeds in a coffee grinder or buy them already ground.

Psyllium. The husk of the psyllium seed forms mucilage that absorbs excess water while stimulating normal bowel elimination.

— **Foods that are excellent sources of fiber include:**

Leafy vegetables: cabbage, lettuce, and spinach.
Stem and squash vegetables: broccoli, cauliflower, asparagus, and celery.
Roots: carrots, beets, and turnips.
Beans and legumes: green beans, soybeans, lentils, pinto, black, red and yellow beans.
Grains: millet, rye, barley, and wild rice.

An increased intake of water and oils will help to reduce constipation. Exercise and intestinal massage also help. Avoid the long-term use of laxatives that stimulate the bowels, such as Senekot or Peri Colace. The body eventually forms a dependence on these stimulants.

Colon hydrotherapy has been used as a method to clean out old stool, which accumulates in the mucosal folds of the colon. The use of colon hydrotherapy can be traced back 2,000 years and is still popular today.

A coffee enema is an effective method for detoxification, mainly because the coffee is absorbed through the intestinal mucosa and goes directly to the liver through the enterohepatic system. It increases the contraction of the bile duct and therefore facilitates excretion of the toxins stored in the gallbladder and bile duct. It is easily done at home. All you need is a pot of organic coffee that has been boiled in filtered water, a simple enema set, and KY jelly or vegetable oil for lubrication. Wait until the coffee reaches room temperature. Lie down on the bathroom floor, insert the tube gently, let the coffee flow in slowly, hold it in as long as you can and massage your abdomen slowly. Evacuate when you need to. Try this the next time you are tired or sick to see whether you feel better afterward. It can be done daily or weekly, depending on the state of your health.

5. The Sweat Pathway of Elimination

Another way the body eliminates toxins is through perspiration. Saunas developed by the Finns and sweat lodges used by Native Americans are good examples of the ways that people recognized the health benefits of sweating. A combination of exercise, vitamins, good nutrition, and regular use of the sauna can dislodge toxins from fatty tissues so that they can then be eliminated from the body by sweating.

If you have access to a sauna in a health club, do aerobic exercise first, take a shower and then sit in the sauna until you sweat. You can take a cold shower and go into the sauna again. Exposure to hot and cold will make the blood vessels dilate and constrict, which helps facilitate the excretion of toxins. If you have an infrared sauna at home, set the temperature from 120° to 140° F and sit in the sauna for 20 to 30 minutes. This will make you sweat profusely. Make sure you drink plenty water to replace the fluid you lose. Combined with exercise and a cold shower, it is a wonderful way to detoxify the body. The difference between an infrared sauna and a health club sauna is that the temperature in an infrared sauna can be adjusted to a lower degree so you can sit there longer, thereby sweating more toxins out of the body.

Finding time to combine your sauna detoxification routine with other daily tasks can be easy and relaxing. I have an infrared sauna at home. I usually bring a book to read, an iPod for my favorite music, a jar of water and a big towel. I set the temperature to 125° F, and after 30 minutes I start to sweat profusely—I can even feel my heart starting to pound faster. When I feel that the sauna has become too hot I will turn it off, but will continue to remain inside for another 10-15 minutes and continue to sweat. This is one of my favorite activities—I get my reading done, toxins sweated out, muscles relaxed, and even get a cardio work out too by increasing my heart rate—all within 45 minutes!

Basic Detoxification—Points to Remember

1. Be aware that we live in a toxic world.
2. Make sure toxin avoidance is your priority.
3. Drink six to eight glasses of water daily.
4. Have one or two bowel movements daily.

5. Sweat regularly by exercising or using a sauna.

6. Regular exercise or lymphatic massage will improve lymphatic flow to help eliminate toxins.

7. Increase your fiber intake by eating more whole grains, nuts, seeds, and vegetables. Supplementation with ground flax seed or psyllium is helpful.

8. Eat high-quality protein, such as eggs or whey protein, to help liver detoxification.

9. Eat at least a cup of cruciferous vegetables (i.e., cabbage, broccoli, kale, cauliflower, Brussels sprouts) daily.

10. Eat celery, onions, grapes, berries, and citrus fruits to help the detoxification process.

11. Use herbs such as cilantro, garlic, ginger, rosemary, turmeric, and curry for detoxification and anti-inflammation actions.

12. Basic supplement for detoxification:

    High-potency multiple vitamin and mineral formula
    Vitamin C (1,000 mg daily)
    Milk thistle (100-200 mg daily)
    Omega-3 fatty acids (1,000-2,000 mg daily)
    Amino acids from whey or egg protein powder (2-4 tablespoons daily)
    Fiber, psyllium or flaxseed fiber (1-2 tablespoons with 8-16 ounces of water daily)

Electromagnetic Frequency (EMF) Contamination

Another potent source of environmental pollution originates from the electromagnetic fields generated by cell phones, power lines, wireless computers, and other electrical devices. Whenever electricity is used or generated, invisible lines of electric and magnetic force are created around its point of origin. Recent studies have raised concerns about the health effects of these electromagnetic frequencies, especially under prolonged exposure. The rapid growth of consumer electronics like cell phones and personal computers have brought the issue of EMF exposure to national attention, and an ever increasing number of national health organizations are recommending caution when it comes to the use of electric devices. To understand the effects of electromagnetic fields on the body, let us take a look at the relationship between electricity and the body's cellular functions.

The body generates its own electricity. That is why we can do an EKG (electrocardiogram) to check a person's heartbeat and an EEG (electroencephalogram) to check their brain waves. Chinese medicine has long called this bioelectricity Chi, our own energy pathway.

When we turn on a light, electricity passes through the wires powering it. The flow of electrons in this circuit creates a magnetic field. When we turn off the light, the flow of electrons ceases and the magnetic field disappears. The greater the light's power, the stronger the magnetic field it creates.

The body will only conduct electricity if the electrical field is strong enough. However, external magnetic fields or electromagnetic frequencies (EMF), such as those generated by electrical systems used to power homes and buildings, can penetrate the body without our awareness whenever we are within reach of that magnetic field. If the body's energy field is affected by this exposure to EMF, cellular functions may also be affected.

We are exposed to EMF contamination from the environment, workplace, and home appliances. Here are some helpful tips and strategies you can employ to help minimize your exposure to EMFs:

- Homes, playgrounds, and schools should be at least 350 feet from high-voltage transmission lines and at least 50 feet from pole-mounted step-down transformers.

- A portable hair dryer can generate high EMF. Keep it away from your head. Wall-mounted hair dryers found in hotels are safer.

- The appliances in kitchens, such as refrigerators, microwaves, electric ovens, dishwashers, juicers, blenders, coffee makers, and toasters can have cumulative effects on EMF. Keep three feet away from these appliances, if possible.

- TVs, CD and DVD players, radios, computers, and printers generate EMF. Keep three feet away, if possible.

- Lights and alarm clocks in the bedroom generate EMF. Keep them at least five feet away from your head.

- Cell phones generate microwaves, just like a microwave oven does. Data concerning the health effects of cell phone-generated microwaves are mounting, but there is currently no consensus on how safe they are. Avoid using your cell phone for an extended period of time. For safety, avoid using your cell phone while you are driving.

Multiple Chemical Sensitivities

Given the large amount of toxic substances in our environment, it is no wonder that many people develop sensitivities and allergies to a number of different chemicals. Yet despite its growing prevalence, this condition is not something that many people are aware of.

Multiple Chemical Sensitivity can best be thought of in this way—imagine that your waste management company has gone on strike, and that garbage has begun to accumulate in your house. The longer the strike, the more the garbage accumulates. The more garbage in your house, the more smelly and dirty your house gets.

It does not matter whether we are exposed to a large amount of toxins all at once, as migrant agricultural workers are with pesticides, or if our bodies accrue small amounts of toxins over an extended period of time due to factors like poor nutrition or mercury leaking from dental fillings. Once we have enough toxins accumulated in the body, we become sick.

Not everyone is affected in the same way because of our genetic differences. These differences affect our capacity to detoxify from chemical substances. Symptoms vary from person to person also, with the most common target organ being the brain. The symptoms of chemical sensitivity can range from fatigue, joint pain, mood swings, brain fog, headaches, dizzy spells, and nausea or flu like illness. Individuals become sensitive and allergic to almost everything. Poor diet, stressful situations, and a lack of sleep and exercise certainly make things worse.

This is a syndrome that frustrates both doctors and patients. Patients who develop multiple chemical sensitivities usually undergo a battery of tests and try multiple medications, only to find that the tests yield no definitive results and the medications make their symptoms worse. It is frustrating for physicians, but even more so for the patients themselves who are tired of being told, "It's all in your head."

There is no standard test physicians can order to confirm the diagnosis. To make things even more confusing, the patients may present multiple symptoms and diagnoses such as fibromyalgia, chronic fatigue syndrome, hypochondria, neurosis, irritable bowel syndrome, chronic insomnia, migraine headaches, neurodegenerative diseases, asthma, hay fever, and auto immune diseases. Many of them have leaky gut syndrome, which opens the gate for toxins getting into our body through the GI tract.

However, there are some tests that may be helpful in determining Multiple Chemical Sensitivities:

- A RBC toxic metal and mineral screen.
- A urine challenge test with DMPS.
- A food allergy test.
- A comprehensive stool analysis.
- Antibodies for candida or wheat.

The treatments are individualized but generally include:

- Toxin avoidance—clean air, clean water, clean house, and clean food.
- Improving nutritional status—avoiding foods the patient is allergic to and replacing healthy bacteria to improve the GI defense mechanism.
- Detoxification with general detox supplements.
- Specific treatments such as IV or oral DMPS chelation for mercury, as well as IV treatments with high doses of the vitamins and minerals that are involved in the liver Phase I and II pathways.

There is no question that we live in a changing environment. The amount of industrial, chemical, and other artificial pollutants contaminating our air, water, and food supply has never been higher, so much so that it is no longer a question of whether we have toxins in our body or not, but how much we can limit the damage that is being done. Nevertheless, even in a toxic world such as ours, it is still possible to experience optimal health and reap the maximum benefit from healing treatments such as bio-identical hormone therapy by reducing our exposure to environmental toxins. Taking positive steps to rid our households of toxic chemicals, improve our nutritional status, and detoxify periodically can make the difference between merely functioning day-to-day and thriving with physical energy, mental clarity, and zest for life!

CHAPTER 12

How to Look 10 Years Younger—Beauty Is Not Just Skin Deep

The Skin

The skin is the largest organ of the body. There are approximately 19 million skin cells on every square inch of the body and the skin keeps renewing itself throughout our lifetime. The pri-mary function of the skin is protection. The skin provides an elastic and waterproof covering to the body to protect it from germs, heat, cold, and the damaging effects of ultraviolet rays in sunlight. The skin has three layers: the epidermis, dermis, and subcutaneous layer.

Skin Structure

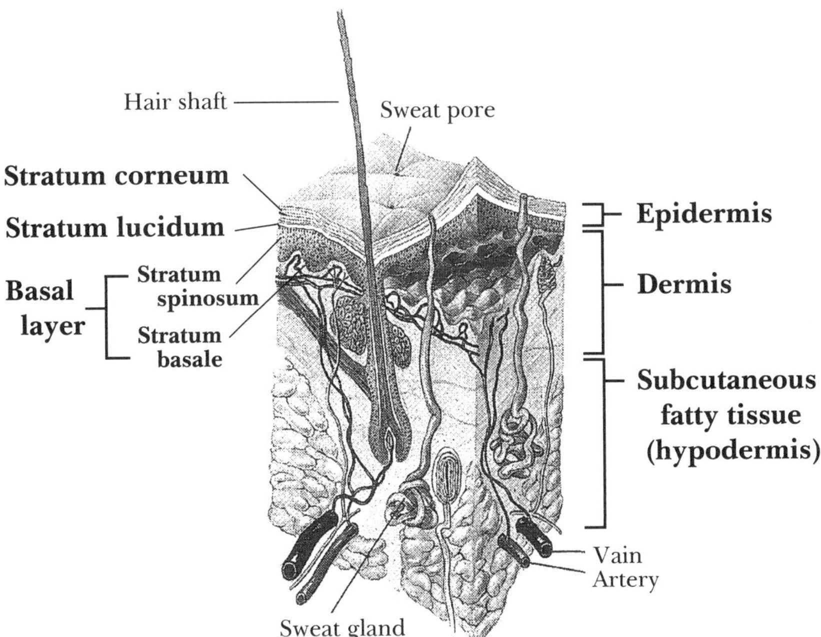

Figure 7.

Epidermis, The Outer Layer

The epidermis has five layers that form the outermost layer of the skin. These layers work together to continually replenish the epidermis in order to form a supple, healthy covering for the body.

- **Stratum corneum**—external layer of the epidermis that holds water inside the body and prevents the entrance of ultraviolet light, pollutants, and chemicals into the body. It is constantly shedding and replenishing itself, completely replacing this layer every month. This process slows down as we get older. Helping this layer shed by using a loofah or body brush will help keep the skin looking younger by removing dead skin cells from the surface.

- **Stratum lucidum** (clear layer)—second layer of the epidermis that consists of small, transparent cells. When the outer layer of cells on the stratum corneum sheds, this layer moves up to become the top layer of the epidermis, which turns over constantly.

- **Stratum granulosum**—exists only in the thick skin found in the palms of the hands and soles of the feet. It helps form a tougher, waterproof barrier to the skin in these areas.

- **Stratum spinosum**–also exists only in the thick skin areas of the body. It provides structural support to help the skin resist abrasion.

- **Stratum basale**—the third layer (fifth layer in hands and feet) of the epidermis generates new epidermal skin cells that will eventually move outward, layer by layer, to become the outermost layer. This deepest layer of the epidermis also contains melanocytes, which produce melanin, a pigment that protects the skin from excessive damage resulting from ultraviolet light. Darker skin results from the production of more melanin. Caucasians have fewer melanocytes, compared to Asians or Africans, which accounts for their lighter skin tone.

Unfortunately, this lack of melanin means there is less protection to the skin from sun damage. Overexposure to ultraviolet sunlight leads to skin cancer and wrinkles. With aging, damaged melanocytes join together, forming pigment blotches that are called sun spots. Malignant melanoma is a cancer of the melanocytes.

Dermis: The Middle Layer

Lying beneath the epidermis, the skin's middle layer is composed of collagen, elastin, and hyaluronic acid, the latter of which holds water. Also embedded in the dermis are blood vessels, lymph vessels, nerve endings, sweat glands, oil glands, and hair follicles.

As skin ages, it loses collagen and elastin. As the body's hormone levels decrease with aging, less oil production occurs for feeding the collagen and elastin. Also with aging, less water retention within the cells results in reduced hyaluronic acid. Both of these impairments lead to the wrinkles that develop in the skin.

Subcutaneous: The Inner Layer

This layer is mainly composed of fat, plus the blood vessels, lymph vessels, and nerves that feed into the dermis. The body loses subcutaneous fat as we age, mostly due to a decline of hormones. This causes the deeper wrinkles, sagging and thinning of the skin.

Skin Damage

The most damaging factor to the skin results from overexposure to sunlight. Other deleterious factors are free radicals that occur as a result of exposure to cigarette smoke, pollutants, harmful bacteria, chemicals, and toxins.

Sun damage causes the skin to develop pigmented blotches; it loses its elasticity and collagen, leading to sun spots, wrinkles and sagginess. If you look at your inner arm versus the side exposed to the sun, you will find that the differences in appearance are all due to sun damage.

The sun's electromagnetic radiation generates three types of ultraviolet (UV) light:

1. **UVA** has the longest wave length and penetrates deeper into the skin layers. This causes tanning of the skin, but it also destroys collagen and elastin in the dermis. Indeed, this UVA light causes the most damage to the skin, yet most tanning salons use this light. It is a slow-reacting light wave and it takes about an hour to get sunburned from exposure to this light.

2. **UVB**, the medium wave length, penetrates less into the skin compared to UVA, but it causes moderate tanning of the skin. It only takes 20 to 30 minutes for UVB to cause sunburn.

3. **UVC** the shortest wave and is rarely heard of because most UVC is filtered out by the earth's ozone layer, therefore exposure only occurs at high altitudes or in areas where the ozone layer is damaged (notably, Antarctica). This very short light wave does not penetrate into the skin deeply, but it can cause sunburn within just one minute of exposure.

Principles of Keeping Your Skin Youthful

Taking steps to protect and nourish your skin is an essential part of every anti-aging plan. Here are the primary rules you should observe in order to keep your skin looking healthy and vibrant for years to come.

- **Avoid sun damage**. Wear a large rim hat with SPF 30 or over. Apply sunscreen to exposed skin to protect yourself from both UVA and UVB. Even on cloudy days, you still need to protect your skin since UV light penetrates through clouds, mist and fog. Avoid exposure to the sun between 10 A.M. and 3 P.M., when UV light is at its strongest. Most sunscreens only work for two hours and some may have harmful chemicals, so you need to use a sunscreen with natural ingredients and antioxidants. Also, be sure to frequently reapply them if you are exposed to the sun continuously or engaged in outdoor activities such as hiking, swimming, or gardening.

- **Hydrate your skin.** The easiest way to hydrate your skin is to drink plenty of water. Additionally, most moisturizers cover and seal your skin to prevent water loss. A mini-facial helps moisturize your skin, such as using a wet towel or steam on your face. Then while the water is still on your skin, seal it with oil such as vitamin E oil.

- **Nourish your skin.** Your skin needs nutrition just like any other part of the body. It is difficult to give nutrition to the skin through a topical cream because the epidermis is a natural barrier. Nonetheless, many capillaries circulate blood just beneath the epidermis, so it is important to get the nutrients that the skin needs through blood circulation. By eating a nutritious diet, you will help to ensure that your skin receives the nutrients it needs. See chapter 9 for details.

- **Keep your hormones levels in the younger age range.** Estrogen increases subcutaneous fat and connective tissue, thus it assists in the prevention of wrinkle formation. Testosterone increases the secretion of oil glands and pre-vents dryness of the skin.

Treatment for Pigmented Skin Blotches and Sun Spots

If your skin is already damaged due to aging and sun exposure, there are steps you can take to repair the damage and keep your skin looking great. In addition to these treatments, be sure to follow the principles for keeping your skin youthful, as discussed above, in order to help maintain your skin's health and appearance.

- Inhibit the formation of melanin (skin pigment) by using creams that contain hydroquinone, kojic acid, or herbs.

- Remove melanin by using Retin-A, skin peel, or laser treatment. Retin-A (or retinol) cream is a form of vitamin A that peels the skin and stimulates growth of the epidermis. Skin peels are usually performed by an aesthetician who applies different chemicals. The beneficial effect of this treatment is limited to the superficial epidermis layer. Laser or light therapy, such as IPL (intense pulsed light), removes deeper epidermal skin layers and also stimulates the formation of collagen.

- Protect new skin by reducing your exposure to the sun.

Treatment for Wrinkles and Sagging Skin

Wrinkles, fine lines and sagging skin resulting from aging and sun damage can also benefit from the following treatments.

- Increase your skin turnover (shedding and replacement of new skin) by using glycolic acid or Retin-A cream.

- Resurface the skin with a facial peel, laser treatment, or IPL (intense pulse light).

- Increase your collagen through laser or IPL treatment. Collagen injections, such as Juvederm or Restylne, can also help to improve suppleness and elasticity.

Laser and IPL

Laser and IPL (intense pulsed light) are light wave treatments for the skin. Different light has varying wave lengths, some of which can reach certain parts of the skin such as pigment layers, hair follicles or blood vessels. Laser has either ablative (removal) or partially ablative abilities. With laser treatment, the superficial layers of the skin can be totally or partially removed. IPL is not immediately ablative; therefore, the skin is not removed at the time of treatment. However, it does cause the skin to peel a few days later. Peeling of the old skin leads to newer and younger skin.

Both treatments can be used to stimulate the formation of collagen and remove pigmented lesions or hairs. These treatments can be combined to achieve better results for skin rejuvenation. Partial skin ablation, such as Fraxel or Pixel Laser treatment, results in less down time for recovery than total skin ablation, such as CO_2 (carbon dioxide) laser or Erbium laser treatment. Partial skin ablation is safer; however, it requires a series of treatments rather than just one treatment. Nonetheless, this approach has grown in popularity since the down time is minimal following treatment.

The side effects of these treatments can be skin irritation; hypopigmentation (loss of skin color), and hyperpigmentation, which causes patches of skin to become darker in color than the surrounding skin. Generally speaking, lighter skin types have fewer complications than individuals with darker skin because with lighter skin there is less pigmentation of skin cells.

After laser or IPL treatment, it is important to follow the recommended skin care program in order to maintain younger-looking skin. Without such a maintenance program, the treated skin will return to its less-than-optimal condition.

Home Skin Care

Great skin care begins at home. In addition to minimizing your sun exposure and eating a balanced-nutritious diet, try the following simple suggestions to supercharge your personal skin care program.

- Avoid sun damage. Use sunscreen with a minimal rating of SPF 15 that includes UVA and UVB protection. Apply each morning before leaving the house. Make sure your sunscreen has natural ingredients, not harsh chemicals, and that it also contains moisturizers and antioxidants. Many sunscreens need to be reapplied every couple of hours. There are a few on the market that last all day. Also, mineral makeup powder has the effect of working as a sunscreen.

- Hydrate your skin at night by steaming your face or putting a wet towel on your face while bathing. Seal the moisture right afterward by massaging vitamin E oil on your face. Spraying your face with thermal spring water periodically throughout the day also helps.

- Use creams that have retinol or glycolic acid daily to stimulate the removal of old skin and the formation of new skin. This will also help the nutrients in the facial cream penetrate into the facial skin.

- Maintain youthful skin by using good skin care products to clean, hydrate, and nourish your skin twice a day. There are two skin care products worth considering. One is vitamin C serum, which is very effective in reducing damage from free radicals—it also provides an anti-inflammatory effect. The other product is spin traps, which are molecules that can catch, hold and deactivate free radicals, thus reducing free radical damage and inflammation of the skin. Regular use of these skin care products can reduce and reverse changes that come with aging skin, such as wrinkles, age spots, and thinning of the skin.

- Do facial treatments regularly, administered either by an aesthetician or yourself. Here is a simple, natural facial you can try at home:

  Before you start: mash ¼ avocado into paste, cut 2 slices of cucumber, put on nice soothing music. Find a chair. Prepare a few hot facial towels.

  Start with washing your face thoroughly with hot water and cleaner, lie down on the floor, put your feet up to a chair, put a hot towel on your face for a few minutes to soften the skin, remove the towel, apply the avocado paste on your face, close your eyes and put a slice of cucumber on each eye. Relax and meditate for 20 minutes.

  Wash off the avocado paste, put a hot towel on your face for a few minutes to increase the moisture on your face, and then do a gentle facial massage. Your face will look wonderful with the oil from avocado, moisture from the hot towel; your facial muscles will be relaxed with the massage and the nice soothing music!

Remember beauty is not just skin deep. Good nutrition and supplements, regular exercise, adequate sleep, stress reduction, maintaining your hormones in good range and reducing toxin exposure are all very important in maintaining your beautiful and healthy skin!

CHAPTER 13

Acupuncture and Herbs—Ancient Chinese Healing

As a physician who emphasizes treatment of the entire body rather than just specific symptoms, I feel that it is important to introduce additional healing modalitics into my patient's routine when I feel that they can provide an appreciable benefit. There is no doubt that treatment with bio-identical hormone pellets can be powerful and life-changing, but sometimes my patients experience additional problems that compound the effects of hormone loss and they do not respond as well to pellets alone. When this occurs, I often recommend treatment with acupuncture and herbs. These healing methods are grounded in ancient traditions and proven in modern practice, which help to enhance the effect of pellet therapy, strengthen internal systems, and assist the body in its restoration to balance. Many patients of mine, like Cynthia, have benefited from this approach.

Cynthia's story:

My name is Cynthia, and even though I was using pellet therapy, Dr. Sun prescribed acupuncture for me. I was going through the pellets quickly, about every three months. Dr. Sun concluded that I was not managing stress well at all. At that time, the stress was job related. I was very aggravated about my work situation and not dealing with it very well. She suggested that I have ten acupuncture treatments.

After the first treatment, I felt better. Even the next day, I could feel that I was more relaxed. What made me a major believer, though, is by the ninth or tenth visit, I had almost a physiological change as a result of the very deep relaxation I experienced from the acupuncture treatments. I was not getting aggravated at all anymore.

I am still at the same job. I can change jobs, but I choose not to do so. Now I have a better perspective on my job. When I become aggravated at work, I take a deep breath, walk out of the office for a few minutes to remove myself from the immediate stress, and remain calm. Now my pellets are lasting between five to six months. I am feeling very well and managing the stress to the point that I am not putting a great deal of strain on my endocrine system.

My body remembers how to relax now, even in stressful situations. But it is not just physical. It is also mental and emotional, which is so important. The acupuncture really changed my human experience related to managing stress. Visiting Dr. Sun is like going to see a physician, therapist, spiritualist, and checking in with your guidance counselor. It is a very holistic and nurturing environment.

Acupuncture is an ancient treatment method that has been practiced for thousands of years. A central component of traditional Chinese medicine, acupuncture's primary aim is to restore and maintain a patient's health through stimulation of key points on the body. Today, physicians often call upon acupuncture as both a primary and complementary treatment for a wide variety of ailments. In my practice, I have been able to witness firsthand the benefits of acupuncture treatment, and when it is appropriate I recommend it to my patients because it simply works. It is not exactly clear, however, as to how it works. Some say it is the result of increased production of endorphins, but I believe that it is due to the balancing of our energy system, which is termed "chi" in Chinese medicine.

A person's body produces its own energy; more precisely, it produces what is termed subtle energy. This energy system is what allows physicians to perform an EKG (electrocardiogram) to detect electric activities in the heart, and an EEG (electroencephalogram) to detect the brain's activities. Akin to the blood vessel system, there is an energy system in the body that is termed the meridian system. Studies have shown that if dyes are injected into certain acupuncture points, they travel to other parts of the body through different paths that have been identified as meridian channels.

According to Chinese medicine, there are twelve meridians: liver, gallbladder, heart, pericardium, triple burner, stomach, spleen, lung, large intestine, urinary bladder, kidney, and small intestine channels. In addition, there are two "master" meridians termed the Du, which means governing in Chinese, and Ren, which means fostering channels.

A basic concept governing Chinese medicine is the Yin (female energy) and Yang (male energy). When Yin and Yang are balanced, the body is in harmony and healthy. This means that if one's energy is balanced and the electric flow throughout the body is smooth, that person feels good and energetic.

Range of Treatment

Acupuncture can be used to treat a wide variety of symptoms and ailments. It is also called upon quite frequently when traditional medications fail to produce results. Here are some of the diseases and conditions that may benefit from acupuncture treatment.

1. Pain Control

This is the most commonly known benefit of acupuncture treatment. Acute and chronic pain, including headache and neck, shoulder, and back pain, are good examples. Other painful conditions associated with arthritis, sports injuries, and post-herpetic neuralgia (shingles) may also be helped by acupuncture treatment.

If effective, acupuncture may be a much better form of treatment than taking pain pills for patients who suffer from chronic pain, because it avoids the deleterious side effects that accompany the chronic use of pain medications.

2. Hormonal Imbalance

Acupuncture combined with herbs has been used for menstrual irregularities, menstrual cramps, premenstrual syndrome, infertility and even menopausal symptoms with some success.

3. Neurological Disorders

Patients suffering from stroke, memory loss and neurodegenerative diseases, such as multiple sclerosis and Parkinson's disease, can stabilize and improve when acupuncture is combined with conventional treatments.

4. Emotional Issues

Acupuncture helps people become more relaxed and calm; as well as helps with anxiety, depression, insomnia, and stress-related conditions. I routinely hear from patients that they sleep better after acupuncture treatment, some even fall into a restful sleep during treatment. It has been widely used for successful treatment of drug or cigarette addiction, probably through reducing craving, anxiety, and depression.

5. Allergies and Autoimmune Diseases

Acupuncture needles inserted in the sinus areas can reduce sinus pressure and inflammation very quickly. Acupuncture combined with herbs can help the body detoxify and improve the immune system. Thus, it can help people with autoimmune diseases.

Fibromyalgia is a disease probably caused by the combination of different triggers such as stress, insomnia, viral infection, hormone loss and imbalance, immune dysfunction, and exposure to toxins. Acupuncture is one of the proven methods of treatment. It probably works by improving sleep, reducing inflammation and pain, and detoxifying the body.

6. Liver Diseases and Digestive Problems

Acupuncture and herbs may improve liver function, constipation, bloating and irritable bowel syndrome.

7. Obesity and Weight Loss

Acupuncture may help people lose weight, probably through reducing cravings, stress reduction and improving detoxification.

Acupressure Points for General Wellness

Like acupuncture, acupressure is an ancient healing art that utilizes the fingers instead of needles to stimulate key points on the body. Acupressure is performed by using your finger to press and rub acupuncture points for one to two minutes. Here are a few acupressure points you can use regularly in the interest of improved health.

Acupressure Points

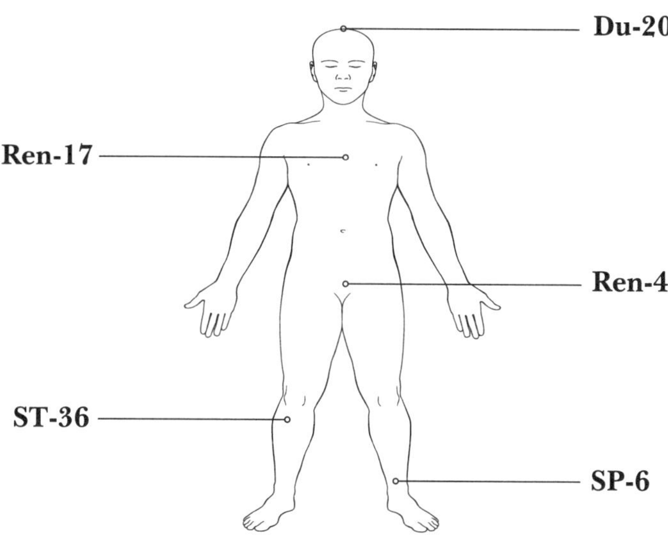

Figure 9. Acupressure points.

- **Du-20.** This is an energy-gathering spot. It is used for toning the Qi (or chi) for the whole body. This point is located on top of the head, where the line between the two ears meets. It correlates to the location of the crown chakra. Tapping this spot may help your brain function better and increase the body's energy level.

- **Ren-17.** This is another energy point located at the mid-line of the chest at the level of the nipples. This is in the same area as the heart chakra. Tapping this point can help to prevent heart and lung diseases as well as boost immunity.

- **Ren-4.** This is another energy point located below the mid umbilicus, close to the second and root chakras. Massaging this point may help digestion, regulate the menstrual period and enhance sexual function.

- **ST-36.** This is one of the most frequently used acupuncture points. It is located about four finger widths below the knee and one finger width from the tibia. Applying acupressure on this point may help digestion, energy and circulation.

- **SP-6.** Three yin meridians (spleen, liver and kidney) all come to this point, which is very important for any women with gynecological disorders but contraindicated during pregnancy. For both men and women, pressing this point may help sexual function, sleep, and digestion.

It takes only ten minutes a day to apply acupressure on these points. If you do it regularly, you will be amazed at how much more energy you will have, along with an increased sense of well-being.

Another approach is to tap each of the meridians from head to toe. You may achieve the same results of increased energy and enhanced well-being by this method as well.

Chinese Herbal Therapy

Herbs are nature's medicine, and have been used in China for thousands of years. This is a time-tested therapy that has proven to be effective and safe, and is still in use today. Herbs play a specific role in Chinese medicine for treating a wide variety of symptoms.

Chinese herbs are not used as a single agent for a certain disease. Rather, they are usually combined to create formulas to treat different diseases and symptoms. This is also time-tested wisdom because the combination of herbs tends to be more effective and to cause fewer side effects.

Herbs of similar actions or different actions are combined together to achieve synergistic effects. There is always one herb added to reduce side effects. This is the unique feature and secret of Chinese formulas. Each ancient formula requires the raw material to be boiled in water to drink as tea. A more modern approach prepares the herbal formulas as pills, powders or in the form of tinctures for convenience of use. Always consult with a trained Chinese medicine doctor before using the formulas in order to achieve the best healing results and to avoid side effects.

For your general well-being, however, the following list provides a few herbs that can be used alone to promote health.

- **Ginseng.** This is the most well known Chinese herb, recognized for its energy boosting qualities. In Chinese medicine, it is used to treat diabetes, heart failure, fatigue and low immunity. In healthy people, it can enhance physical and mental well-being. Ginseng is an adaptogen (a class of herbs that helps the body adapt to stressful situations) and is very useful for the treatment of adrenal fatigue and hormone imbalance. Three types of ginseng are available on the market: Korean red ginseng, Chinese ginseng, and American ginseng. If you have high blood pressure, using Korean red ginseng may elevate your blood pressure even more; then Chinese ginseng is a better choice.

- **Goji** (Lycium berries). Like other berries, goji is plentiful in antioxidants and phytochemicals (plant-derived chemical compounds that provide healing benefits). In Chinese medicine, it is used for anti-aging, as well as treating menopausal symptoms and improving blurred vision. Currently it is very popular, and you can find goji drinks everywhere. Chinese cuisine uses dried goji in different soups, making them very tasty.

- **Dong quai** (Chinese angelica root). Dong quai is an herb famous for its benefits to the female reproductive system. It has a rich supply of phytochemicals and has been used to treat menstrual problems. It is also used as an anti-aging herb.

- **Juhua** (Chrysanthemum). Juhua is used both as a food and a medicinal herb in China. Juhua green tea is used to treat the flu and to help diminish symptoms of cough and sore throat. Like goji, juhua may also improve eye function.

The difference between Chinese medicine and orthodox Western medicine is that Chinese medicine does not target one organ. Instead, it treats the entire body and aims for balance of the body's energy to facilitate its own healing power. Also,

Chinese medicine's main emphasis is on the prevention of diseases and the treatment is highly individualized. This is why the practitioner's experience and intuition are very important in attaining optimal treatment results. The effects of acupuncture and herbs are usually not as dramatic as those achieved in Western medicine, but the side effects profile is much better.

Acupuncture and herbal treatment are not contradictory to Western medicine. As a matter of fact, they can be complementary to each other. While Western medicine is more advanced in diagnostic tools and surgeries, Chinese medicine is better at preventing diseases and promoting the body's own healing systems. Integrating both of these approaches can often produce the best results. If orthodox Western medicine can modify its direction of treatment from a single disease to the whole person, focus more on prevention instead of treating illness, and tailor treatment programs that recognize a patient's individuality, then everyone stands to benefit—the practice of medicine will be advanced through an integrative approach that provides doctors with the tools they need to help patients become happier and healthier.

CHAPTER 14

Our Mind—You Are What You Think

In this chapter, we are going to explore the science of the mind-body connection and the potential it has to help us heal in ways we would never have thought possible.

The Mind—Body Connection

Think of our body as a computer. If the brain is the hardware, the mind is the software. The brain controls the body through hormones and neurotransmitters; the mind governs the brain with thoughts and feelings. Together, they rule our behavior, emotions, and the many different functions of our body. Everything we do starts from the mind. It is extremely powerful, and it can make you or break you!

Let us look at how the mind exerts its influence. If you simply think, for example, of eating a lemon, without even seeing the lemon you start to secrete saliva just by thinking about how sour it is. Or if you receive a letter from the IRS (Internal Revenue Service), your mind races even before you have opened the letter as you wonder if the IRS plans to audit you. Your heart pounds a little faster and anxiety arises. After you open the letter and discover the IRS is going to refund you a few thousand dollars, your heartbeat slows down again and you feel happy knowing that you will not be facing an ordeal.

It is estimated that over half of the office visits to family practitioners or general internists are due to emotionally related physical symptoms. If the physician focuses on the illness without paying attention to the underlying emotional cause, that illness will probably not improve much, and additional emotionally driven illnesses will probably also occur.

The Brain

The human brain has three parts: the forebrain, midbrain, and hindbrain. The forebrain contains lobes of the cerebral cortex that control higher functions, such as thinking, reasoning, and speaking. The midbrain and hindbrain control the unconscious autonomic functions of the body. Specific behaviors are associated with different parts of the brain.

- **The Cerebrum**

  The cerebrum, the evolutionary new part of the human brain, is divided into symmetric left and right hemispheres. Within these hemispheres are the prefrontal and frontal cortex, temporal lobes, basal ganglia, occipital lobes, hypothalamus, and the pituitary glands.

  — The frontal lobes are divided into three parts:

    - the motor cortex, which controls movement such as walking
    - the premotor cortex, which involves the planning of motor movement
    - the prefrontal cortex, which coordinates planning, organization impulse control, and communication.

    The prefrontal cortex is the most evolved part of a human being. It is what makes humans stand out from other animals. This is the part of the brain from which anxiety and worry emanate.

    If this part of the brain works right, a person is organized, thoughtful, empathetic, and communicative. They can learn from mistakes and make plans to reach goals. When it does not work adequately, it results in poor judgment, a short attention span, trouble learning from experience, poor time management, or difficulty with organization to perform tasks.

— The temporal lobes lay at the sides of the brain and are involved with the subconscious mind. The functions carried on here are:

- short-term memory and memory storage
- language and auditory (hearing) processing
- storage of remembered feelings and emotions

Problems in the temporal lobes lead to memory loss, learning and reading difficulties, difficulty with speech, or unstable moods. This is the first area damaged by Alzheimer's disease.

— The basal ganglia area is involved with:

- motor control
- cognition
- emotions
- learning

Low activity in this area, such as in Parkinson's disease, leads to slow movement, tremors, and problems with writing, walking, and other daily activities.

Other diagnoses linked to injured basal ganglia include, among others, ADHD (attention deficit hyperactivity disorder), cerebral palsy, obsessive-compulsive disorder, and stuttering.

— The occipital lobes are located in the back of the skull. It is the visual processing center where everything that we see is interpreted, analyzed, and integrated with the other parts of the brain.

— Hypothalamus and pituitary glands. The hypothalamus secretes hormones to regulate the pituitary gland. Located at the bottom of the brain, the pituitary gland hangs like a little pearl into its own small, protective skull pocket. It secretes growth hormone along with other hormones that control the thyroid and adrenal glands, as well as the ovaries or testes.

- **The Cerebellum**

The cerebellum, also called the small brain, is the older part of the brain. Even though its size represents only 10 percent of the brain, it contains 50 percent of the brain's neurons or nerve cells. Located at the bottom of the brain, it is the major motor coordination center. Problems in this part of the brain result in poor handwriting, or being clumsy or accident-prone.

Neurotransmitters and the Neuroendocrine Communication System

Neurotransmitters are the chemical messengers that have either inhibitory or excitatory functions. If the neurotransmitters are balanced, the brain will be balanced. Too much stimulatory neurotransmitters or not enough inhibitory neurotransmitters will make a person nervous or anxious, while the opposite leads to depression or other problems.

There are six major neurotransmitters:

- Neuro-excitatory: epinephrine (adrenaline), norepnephrine, glutamate.
- Neuro-inhibitory: serotonin, GABA (gamma-aminobutyric acid).
- Both excitatory and inhibitory: dopamine.

Acetylcholine is another neurotransmitter that is typically involved with memory.

- **Serotonin**

Serotonin is the most well-known and studied neurotransmitter because many antidepressant medications, such as Prozac, Zoloft, and Paxil, are selective serotonin reuptake inhibitors (SSRIs). This means that these medications increase the level of serotonin to relieve depression. All neurotransmitters are made from amino acids, so if the intake of the precursor amino acids is increased, neurotransmitters will also increase.

The amino acid tryptophan converts to 5 HTP (5-hydroxy-tryptophan), which then converts to serotonin. This neurotransmitter further converts to melatonin, which is the hormone that helps regulate sleep.

When serotonin is low, norepinephrine or dopamine may be over expressed, resulting in the fight-or-flight response and leading to panic attacks and anxiety. Low levels of serotonin lead to low melatonin, which causes insomnia. Low serotonin levels are also associated with PMS (premenstrual syndrome), eating disorders, migraine headaches, and depression.

- **GABA**

GABA (gamma-aminobutyric acid) is a neuro-inhibitory neurotransmitter. Low levels of GABA lead to insomnia, irritability, anxiety and panic attacks. Amino acids, such as theanine and taurine, increase the functions of GABA, as do tranquilizers and alcohol.

- **Dopamine**

Dopamine has both an inhibitory and excitatory function. It increases the secretion of growth hormone (GH) by increasing GH-releasing hormone, and plays a major role in motor function, memory, cognition, and focus.

Dopamine deficiency can result in attention deficit disorder (ADD), poor memory, and motor dysfunction, as seen in Parkinson's disease. Low levels of dopamine also mean low levels of pleasure. The SSRI (selective serotonin reuptake inhibitor) group of antidepressants inhibits dopamine function, which helps to explain why people on antidepressants may have low libido, or be emotionally flat.

- **Epinephrine, Norepinephrine, and Glutamate**

  Epinephrine, norepinephrine, and glutamate are all excitatory neurotransmitters. Epinephrine (adrenaline) is the principle hormone produced by the adrenal glands. It travels through the blood stream to the brain. Another source of epinephrine occurs from the conversion of norepinephrine in the presence of cortisol. These hormones have excitatory functions and have to be balanced with inhibitory neurotransmitters in order for individuals to function well.

Brain Health and Hormones

Hormones have a deep impact on the brain because they are essential players in the fundamental communication of billions of nerve cells. In their roles as regulators and stimulators, hormones are responsible for brain functions that determine mood status, memory storage, cognitive capacities and sexual desires. Let us take a look at each one of them:

- **Estrogen**

  — Increases the amount of mood regulating neurotransmitters, including norepinephrine, serotonin, and also acetylcholine, which improves memory.

  — Increases the density of neurotransmitter receptors on the cell membrane of neurons, which helps improve the functioning of the neurotransmitters.

  — Increases the growth and survival of nerve cells. Estrogen deficiency may lead to brain atrophy and death of nerve cells.

  — Increases the ability of neurons to connect in various part of the brain, regulating emotional states such as depression and anxiety.

  — Is necessary for blood flow to the parts of brain that are responsible for emotion, memory and cognitive functions.

- **Progesterone**

  — Is involved in mood and memory, but through a different pathway than estrogen.

  — Can counterbalance and offset some of the effects of estrogen on mood and memory.

  — Increases GABA levels by converting to allopregnenolone, which is one of the most potent modulators of GABA receptors in brain cells. By increasing the calming neuro transmitter GABA, progesterone helps women relax and sleep better.

- **Testosterone**

  — Influences the areas of brain that regulate sexual responsiveness. It increases libido and is a powerful treatment for sexual dysfunction in both men and women.

  — Influences cognitive function, and improves both learning and memory.

  — Improves the mood and can work as an effective antidepressant, without the side effects of antidepressant medications.

- **Thyroid Hormone**

  It is well known that depression can be the result of low thyroid hormone. Thyroid hormones regulate metabolism for the whole body and if thyroid hormones are low, nothing works right. Depression, irritability, memory loss and brain fog are common symptoms when thyroid is low.

- **Cortisol**

  Excessive cortisol (cortisone) inhibits serotonin through different mechanisms at receptor sites in brain cells. Cortisol also converts norepinephrine to epinephrine. When this happens, external stress can lead to increased anxiety or depression.

In summary, 5-HTP, thyroid hormone, estrogen and testosterone all boost serotonin function. Progesterone improves GABA levels. Estrogen and testosterone both improve acetylcholine levels, and the blood circulation to the brain, thus they improve memory and slow down brain aging.

In my practice, I have been able to gradually reduce and then discontinue use of antidepressants for many of my patients, once estradiol and/or testosterone pellet implants have begun to work. I also use bio-identical progesterone, either in the form of cream, lozenges or pills in women who suffer from PMS, insomnia, anxiety, and moodiness with good results.

When we treat mood issues in menopausal women or andropausal men, hormone treatment should be the first choice, not antidepressants or tranquilizers. Reducing stress hormones and optimizing the thyroid hormone can also contribute significantly to the improvement of mood and cognitive functions of the brain.

The neuroendocrine system is very complex. It involves neurons, neurotransmitters, hormones, carrier proteins and receptors. Treatments that help balance neurotransmitters and hormones are the keys to optimal health.

How to Improve Brain Health

Brain cells, like other cells in the body, need balanced hormones, adequate nutrition and oxygen, as well as avoidance of exposure to toxins. Here are ways to help maintain good health for the brain:

- Brain cells do not repair as easily as cells in other organs. In fact, until recently, it was believed that brain cells could not even regenerate. Precautions should always be taken to minimize the risk of head injuries. Always wear a helmet when riding a bicycle or motorcycle. Do not participate in dangerous sports. Always wear a seat belt. By all means, do not drink and drive.

- Aerobic exercise brings more blood to the brain, which results in more oxygen and nutrients.

- Specific brain exercises will build new transmission pathways and enhance brain function. Learning to do new things is a form of mental exercise. Music, dance, reading books, creative writing or doing crossword puzzles are all good examples of brain exercises.

- Balanced and optimized hormones such as estrogen, testosterone, progesterone, and thyroid hormones are very important for the brain to function well.

- Stress reduction is important because high levels of cortisol and adrenaline (epinephrine) interfere with brain function.

- A high protein and low-carbohydrate diet is essential for a healthy brain because neurotransmitters are made from amino acids, which are derived from protein. High or low levels of sugar will adversely affect the brain's capacity to work.

- Avoid stimulants like caffeine, as they worsen anxiety. Alcohol's depressive function on the brain also interferes with optimal brain health.

- Good fat, especially DHA (docosahexaenoic acid) from omega-3 fatty acids, is a building block for cell membranes of the brain. It also protects the brain by reducing inflammation.

- Supplements such as 5-HTP and SAMe (S-adenosyl-L-methionine) increase the body's level of serotonin. Melatonin helps with sleep. Many antioxidants help prevent brain aging.

The Conscious, Subconscious, and Unconscious Mind

The majority of the mind is unconscious, and is formed during the first few years of life. The conscious mind is just the tip of the iceberg. Between the conscious and unconscious levels of the mind is the subconscious, which can be brought to conscious awareness when an individual is deeply relaxed.

The unconscious mind is made of suppressed memories and remembered feelings from early childhood. Its impressions are established very early in life. These impressions are carried throughout a person's lifetime without that person knowing much about its content.

A person can have a panic attack, for example, and never know what brought on the feeling of dread that triggered the episode. Or someone can go into an uncontrollable rage in reaction to a very minute incident. Or an individual can be attracted to another person without really knowing why. Or a person cannot control eating habits, even though that person knows not to over eat.

These are examples of when we know at a conscious level that we should or should not do certain things, but mental blocks in the subconscious or unconscious hold us back.

The distinction between the unconscious level of mind and the subconscious is a fine line. We can access the subconscious mind when we reduce conscious control through meditation or hypnosis. We can screen our thoughts consciously in an attempt to figure out what the subconscious is telling us.

The mind is largely composed of the thoughts, feelings, sensations and behavioral feedback that emanate from all of its levels—the conscious, subconscious and unconscious. If we can better understand what is going on in the subconscious and unconscious levels, we can train our conscious mind to reduce negative thoughts and to develop positive thoughts instead. We can also tap into our subconscious mind for creativity and unleash the massive potential that is innate to our being. In other words, by working to integrate these three levels of the mind, the outcome can be wondrously improved. We do not have to stay stuck in patterns of thinking, feeling and behaving.

How does one tap into the subconscious, and open the hidden power of our mind? Meditation, creative visualization, positive affirmation and self-hypnosis are all important tools.

Meditation

Meditation is the act of letting your mind become quiet and removing noisy thoughts from your conscious level. As you relax and the mind becomes quiet, you will be able to connect to your subconscious.

Just like a glass of sandy water, the mind is murky when all of its particles have been swirling in response to the day's stressors and demands. But if you let the glass of sandy water sit for awhile, the sand will settle down at the bottom and the water will become clear. This is the way that meditation clears the mind.

Meditation is one of the most important tools you have to tap into the treasures of your subconscious mind. As valuable as it is, however, meditation can be very difficult to do. I have been trying for many years and still feel I have a long way to go.

Meditation can be performed in an extended session of 20 to 45 minutes, or a short session that can take less than five minutes.

Three Phases of Meditation

1. **Intention**

   Always know what you want to accomplish before meditation. For instance, you may want to be calmer or more relaxed, or you may want to solve a problem you are facing, or you may want to improve your relationship with someone.

2. **Execution**

   Once you have focused on your intention, then stop thinking and allow the body to relax and the mind to become focused on letting go of daily concerns. Several techniques, listed below, can help in achieving this.

3. **Reflection**

   At the end of the meditation, remain quiet and recall any experiences from the session that stands out in your mind. This will reinforce the mental process related to your goal.

Four Meditating Techniques

1. Centering

The centering technique maintains continuous awareness of something, such as focusing on your breathing in the abdominal area. Centering helps your mind to focus. Just like a boat that has been anchored, the mind does not stay still, but after drifting a little, the anchor holds it back. Do not be dismayed when thoughts interrupt your focus. Simply return to the process of focusing on your breathing. As long as you keep bringing your awareness back to your center after your mind has drifted a little, you are on the right track.

2. Attending

The attending technique builds on centering. During centering practice, you ignore distractions. During attending practice, you identify distractions and then disengage from them and go back to centering. If the distractions keep returning, simply saying "later" in your mind will help. This technique will help you become more open and aware to what is going on inside you and will help you build a mind that is flexible and tolerant.

3. Concentrating

When you practice concentrating, you focus intently on a mental object. First, observe a simple physical object such as a key or an apple. Then close your eyes and allow the memory of the object to appear in your mind. If you lose track of the mental image of the object, simply refresh your mind by observing the object again. Repeat the last two steps until you can focus clearly on the mental image of that object. Mastering this technique helps to develop creative visualization and the imagination. This technique could also sharpen your mind.

4. Opening

Opening is a meditative technique that develops spaciousness. It is like being in a boat, then suddenly becoming a fish swimming in the ocean, or becoming a bird and flying away. A sense of freedom and joy comes with it. No matter what is going on with your body, your mind can still soar. To do a brief opening session, simply envision a sense of space or vastness. Then inhale deeply, pretending that there is space inside your body and the inhaled air is filling it. As you release your breath, imagine that all the things that bother you are moving out of your body into the space surrounding you and moving away distantly. This technique is the most advanced since it builds on centering, attending, and concentrating. Spaciousness is a key to tapping creativity, finding solutions, and experiencing more joy and less worry. This is also the most useful technique for solving problems and achieving peace and joy.

Brief meditation is easy to do for those who feel they do not have the time to do an extended meditation. It can be done for a few minutes before falling to sleep or upon awakening in the morning. It can be done while you are in the shower or waiting in line. It can even be done when you are walking. You can do brief meditation a few times a day. Before long, you will be ready to do extended meditation with similar techniques, except that you will need a certain amount of time without interruption.

Steps for Creative Visualization and Positive Affirmations

- Sit comfortably in a chair or on the floor or lie on a bed and close your eyes.

- Take a deep breath; inhale and exhale slowly; relax your body.

- Count down from 50 to 1. Relax your body from head to toe progressively by first contracting and then relaxing the muscles in your neck, face, eyes and jaw. Then move gradually downward as you relax your shoulders, arms, hands, fingers, back, belly and hips, moving further downward toward your thighs, calves, ankles and lastly your feet and toes.

- Now that your body is relaxed, start the creative visualization and positive affirmations. Repeat them mentally. Here are examples of positive affirmations:

  I am calm, I am relaxed.
  I am confident, I am at peace.
  I am kind, I am compassionate.
  I am healthy, I am attractive.
  I maintain a healthy body and mind, and I always do so.

Combining Positive Affirmations with Visualization

- Examples

Creative visualization, positive affirmations, and self-hypnosis are very similar. Combined with meditation, they can become powerful tools to reshape your mind and change your life. As little as ten minutes a day will do wonders if you are persistent!

— Visualize yourself playing tennis. You run smoothly, arriving just in time to accurately hit the ball with a crisp sound.

— Visualize yourself giving a presentation. You walk into a room full of people, greet them, smile, and begin your presentation with confidence, calmness and articulate clarity.

— Visualize the fat in your abdominal area melting away.

— Visualize a laser gun destroying a tumor in your body.

— Remember the happiest moment in your life. Play it back like a movie, recalling the sights, sounds and feelings associated with the memory. Remember any particular smells, the taste of certain foods and the touch of different objects and people.

— Imagine your goal has been achieved. Sense the sights, savor the sounds; recall the smells and remember feelings that accompany this success.

— Visualize a golden ray of energy coming into your body through your feet, moving upward along your thighs, pelvis, stomach, heart and lungs, and brain. This golden light brings a flood of energy, healing every part of your body.

You can design the visualization to suit your needs to best accomplish any goal you wish to achieve.

— Say to yourself: "I am going to count from one to five. When I reach five, I will open my eyes, feeling fine and better than before."

— At the count of five, open your eyes and affirm mentally, "I am wide awake, feeling fine and better than before."

Once we learn how to tap into our subconscious mind, the next step is to do an honest assessment of ourselves, our self esteem and how to improve it. Developing people skills and learning how to relate to one another is also very important, as most problems we encounter in life start from relationship issues.

Self-esteem

Self-esteem is how we see and value ourselves. Typically, this is the result of remembered feelings that have originated from childhood experiences that carry through to adulthood. It is the self-image formed as an individual internalizes feedback from the environment.

A person who was raised in a negative environment as a child and was constantly criticized or punished would predictably have low self-esteem, even if extremely intelligent. Worst of all, when that person grows up, the subconscious and unconscious will continue the pattern of criticism to which that person has become accustomed. Low self-esteem can lead to failure in school, work and social interactions. Past failures will further lower one's self-esteem, which will only lead to more failures in the present. This then becomes a vicious cycle of ongoing self-defeat.

Low self-esteem often leads to depression or anxiety, or both. It is also a major reason people do not reach their full potential. To build self-esteem, you need to do an honest evaluation of yourself, recognizing that everybody has strengths and weaknesses.

Inflated self-confidence can be just as bad. If you overestimate your ability and the world around you does not provide support, you will be subject to disappointment and frustration. In addition, grandiose ideas lead to a sense of entitlement and arrogance. These handicaps make it difficult to build satisfying relationships.

Implanting positive thoughts and emotions through creative imagination and self-hypnosis are very effective ways to not only improve self-esteem but to help a person achieve their life ambitions. It is like planting more flowers in the field to make it a lovely place to enjoy. Psychotherapy is for people who need extra help. It helps a person to understand the dysfunctional patterns established in early childhood. Restructuring feedback and self-awareness skills will help repair the negative self-image from these early stages of development. It is like pulling the weeds from a field so we can have room to plant more flowers.

Ways to Examine and Build Your Self-esteem

1. Write down three of your strengths.

2. Write down three things you have accomplished that make you proud of yourself.

3. Write down three things you can reward yourself for that do not involve money or food.

4. Write down three things you can do to make yourself feel good and three more things you can do to make others feel good.

5. Write down three things you want to improve about yourself and how you will accomplish them.

Relationships and People Skills

Most problems in life are due to troubled relationships. If we have good people skills, we can avoid many of these problems. With a support system of family and friends, achieving success and happiness become much easier.

Important People Skills

- Communication skills. Communication involves the ability to understand another person and the ability to express yourself and be understood. To understand other people, you have to listen and put yourself in the other person's shoes. This is the way to develop a sense of empathy. To be understood, you have to know what you want and how to express yourself clearly. Communication is the basis for all relationships. If there is no two-way communication, the relationship suffers. Bad communication leads to a bad relationship. The book Men Are from Mars and Women Are from Venus, by John Gray, illustrates how men and women think differently, which creates more challenges in communication. Communication builds on the understanding of yourself and another person.

- Think before you talk. Be positive and polite. Do not criticize, especially if you are angry. We often say things when we are angry that we later regret. Besides, we usually do not get what we want when we criticize. Remember, only honey attracts bees.

- Do not avoid dealing with conflict. This will only lead to frustration, depression or withdrawing from the relationship. When dealing with difficult issues or conflicts, try to remain objective and to not get emotional. Stand up for yourself without being angry. Be kind but firm. Act, do not react.

Important Points on Building Positive Relationships

- Always be honest and trustworthy. Lies are eventually discovered. When that happens, trust evaporates. When people discover they have been cheated, the relationship is broken, sometimes irretrievably.

- Never take a relationship for granted. This happens in marriage quite often and becomes a problem when the husband or wife does not respect or appreciate what their mate is doing for them. Gratitude goes a long way toward keeping the love in a relationship vibrant.

- Be thoughtful and considerate. A selfish person or self-centered person is difficult to deal with a lot of the time. Make sure the relationship is a win-win situation for both individuals.

- Take responsibility for any unpleasant situation. A relationship is not a one-way street. You play a role, too. Do not just blame the other person. Look at developing the ability to establish boundaries, and then communicate them clearly so that the other person can learn what is important to you.

- Do not spread gossip or criticize other people when they are not around. It is much better to confront the other person directly and resolve the issue.

- Keep your promises. Do not make a promise if it is unlikely that you can keep it.

Be assertive and kind. Do not be aggressive or passive, both can lead to resentment. Take a risk on letting the other person know what you need. Learn how to accept defeat graciously and how to win with humility. Above all, be lovable and seek ways to make the other person in the relationship happy. Such positive behavior is generally reciprocated.

Mental Exercises: Training for Happiness and Positive Thinking

Positive thinking that leads to happiness is a choice. It does not require money, fame, or success as a prerequisite. A person does not even need a perfect body or perfect mate to be happy. It can start right now by simply choosing it.

During World War II, Dr. Viktor Frankl, a psychiatrist and a Jew, was imprisoned by the Nazis in Auschwitz, a concentration camp located in German-occupied southern Poland. His parents, brother, and wife all died in the camp. Frankl himself suffered torture and innumerable indignities. One day, naked and alone in his small room, he formulated his theory, called "the last human freedom." It was a freedom within himself that not even his Nazi captors could take away from him. They could completely control his environment, they could do what they wanted to his body, but he alone could decide how all of these atrocities would affect him. While he could not control what happened to him, he had total freedom and the power to choose his response.

Dr. Frankl, by using his mind power and self-discipline, survived the torture and became an inspiration to those around him, including the prison guards. After being released from the concentration camp, he wrote *Man's Search for Meaning*, which depicts the horrors of that experience and how his philosophy on the ultimate freedom to interpret the meaning of life experiences helped him to survive.

In our daily lives, we have many stressors and worries. Your spouse may have a different point of view on important family issues that leads to disagreements or fights; your children may not be doing well in school; your parents may be sick and need you to care for them; your job may be more demanding of your time and attention than you can give; that stack of bills just keeps piling higher and higher. Anger, worry, anxiety and depression are common reactions to these situations. But you do have a choice regarding how you will respond to these stressors, with thoughts and emotions that are either positive or negative in nature.

At the center of this choice is the realization that it is you and not anyone else who can make you happy, in spite of life's challenges and difficulties. Training for happiness has two parts:

1. Identify and cultivate a positive mental state. This includes peace, serenity, calm, love, forgiveness and compassion.

2. Identify and eliminate a negative mental state. This includes depression, anxiety, anger, hatred, worry and guilt.

We all know that the glass can be half full or half empty. It is also true that things can look differently if we look at them from a variety of perspectives. The Chinese word "crisis" actually incorporates two words: danger and opportunity. Even in a crisis, there is an opportunity to make things better or to become a better person.

Depression is anger turned inwardly upon yourself, usually when you are not happy with yourself or your situation. You may feel trapped. The way out of depression is to realize that you are not trapped. You do have alternative choices. It is simply a matter of discovering them and making the best choice within the bounds of your control. After all, it is a sense of control that is often at the base of personal happiness.

Anxiety occurs when you do not know how to handle a situation. It is at times such as this that you have the opportunity to build your self-esteem and learn skills to handle issues with relationships,

Anger only leads to hatred and destruction. There is no justified anger. The challenge is to do something constructive about the things you do not like. One example is MADD (Mothers against Drunk Drivers), which was created when a mother lost her child due to a drunk driver. She turned her anger into a proactive way to prevent drunk driving, car accidents and fatalities.

Worry is forecasting the future and anticipating that something bad will happen. While worry can help us prepare for a coming event, when carried to an excess, it becomes counterproductive. This provides an opportunity to improve a poor self-image or low self-esteem as well as to learn how to not become too attached to the outcome of a situation.

Guilt is living in the past, regretting what you have done. If you truly have regret, apologize sincerely, pay the consequences, forgive yourself and see this as a learning experience so you do not make the same mistake again.

Changing your thoughts from negative to positive will reward you with a positive mental state. The techniques of meditation, creative visualization, positive affirmations, and self-hypnosis will help tremendously in making this mental switch. If you are unable to handle this task yourself, try working with a mental health professional for marriage and family counseling, psychotherapy, or psychoanalysis, which can be very effective. Denial will not solve problems. It only leads to more problems. Taking a proactive stance by confronting difficult situations—internally or in the external environment—is always rewarded with progress and lays the groundwork for happiness and good health.

CHAPTER 15

Spirit—You Are What You Believe

The inner space inside
That we call the heart
Has become many different
Living scenes and stories.

A pasture for sleek gazelles,
A monastery for Christian monks,
A temple with Shiva dancing,
A Kaaba for pilgrimage.

The tablets of Moses are there
The Qur'an, the Vedas,
The sutras and the gospels.
Love is the religion in me.

Whichever way love's camel goes,
That way becomes my faith,
The source of beauty, and the light
Of sacredness over everything.

—Rumi (1207-1273)

Have you thought about 100 years from now, when almost everybody who is alive now will be dead?

Have you thought about 200 years from now, when most of the buildings that exist today will be destroyed, rebuilt or in ruin?

Have you thought about the differences between humans and other animals?

Have you thought about the purpose of our life?

I am not a theologian or philosopher, but years of medical practice and seeing thousands of people in various life stages has given me the chance to peek into life on our world through a special scope. I have found that as a physician I can treat illness, but true healing is beyond medical treatment. It has to do with our mind and spirit, that mystical place within us.

I have found that many people who have money and power are not necessarily happy or content with their lives. The people who seem to be happiest are those who are spiritual, kind, appreciative and loving. Their financial status or material achievements have not made them who they are. Rather, they have achieved their successes in life as a result of their caring and compassionate nature and high ethical standards.

Many people seem to be struggling with day-to-day life; they seem to have no system of belief to help them tackle obstacles and make progress. So, they always seem to end up back at square one, frustrated, never certain why they are so stuck, and not knowing for sure how to get unstuck.

Earlier in my life, I was like that, too. After I reached 50, a light bulb turned on in my head. I realized that I was getting older and would not be around forever. I pondered the purpose and meaning of my life. I looked back and saw that the harder I had worked the more struggles I had to face. I questioned what would happen to me at the end of my life. I reached out for spiritual answers to my life issues.

God must have heard me because, since that time, different people have shown up in my life to lead me on the spiritual path. I will always be a truth seeker, and I would like to share with you what I have discovered so far.

Philosophy of Life

Your belief system defines what is in your mind, what kinds of choices you make, what you do with your life and how you treat other people in your life. Just as the operating system and applications software of a computer determine how the hardware functions, your belief system shapes your philosophy toward life and the way you will live. The end result is that it molds you into the kind of person you are now and will become in the future.

These beliefs or attitudes cover a wide spectrum of human behavior. Non-selfishness, detachment from the material world, appreciating the present moment, observance of the laws of cause and effect, how to obtain true happiness, understanding the value of affliction and suffering, the ability to forgive and love, and the acceptance of others, are powerful concepts that help shape your life into a meaningful experience. These qualities are not only beneficial to yourself, but they help you to be supportive of others, who also are learning how to live in balanced ways through skillful use of their power of free will.

Purpose of Life: Service, Not Self-centeredness

When I first read *The Purpose-Driven Life* by Rick Warren, I did not like it. What was he insinuating when he said, "We were planned for God's pleasure?" Was he asserting that I have to give up my own will to be a slave to God? But little by little, I have discovered the value of his perspective.

We create our own suffering by putting ourselves at center stage, with our egos and self-absorptions as the main attractions. We worry if we do not have enough money. We get angry when things do not go our way. We get depressed when we do not have what we want.

What if we take ourselves out of center stage and put God there instead? Judaism and Christianity tell us to love God and to love our neighbors as ourselves. I believe that human beings are created by God, and that God knows what humans need to be happy and prosperous. Why then do we not search for God's way as we conduct the business of our lives? A God-centered existence creates meaning and purpose in all that we do in this world.

A Chinese proverb says: "Against heaven's rules, you will be extinguished. Following heaven's rules, you will prosper." If we live by spiritual principles, God gives us all that we need, which is primarily love, and that love inspires us to give to others what we have so freely received.

We discover then that the purpose of our lives is to serve not ourselves, but our families, our neighbors, our society, and God.

Living in such a way as to be helpful and of service to those in need around us carries within itself the seeds of soul satisfaction and self-respect.

Imagine a society in which big business does not focus solely on profit, but also on the well-being of its workers. Imagine companies selling products that help instead of damage the environment. Imagine politicians who are not persuaded by influential lobbyists and donors, but who focus on what is best for their constituents and society in general. Imagine a society that takes care of the elderly, the young, the sick, and the helpless instead of catering only to wealthy and healthy individuals. Imagine a society that has no crime, violence, or illegal drugs. Imagine a society in which all people live together peacefully, where all take pride in doing their jobs well, and all are happy. Imagine countries that do not go to war in order to fight over different belief systems or for abuse of power.

We all have different talents that God has given us. We just need to find them and use them over the course of our lives. This will make us passionate, creative, happy, and productive. In such purpose-driven individuals, there is no room for low self-esteem, self-pity, fear, anger, depression and anxiety.

A life without purpose is like a ship without a compass or driving without a map. Many people focus only on money and pleasure, which may bring temporary happiness but are never fulfilling in themselves. Money is neutral, and when used to foster the well-being of others, it can be very fulfilling. Such a purpose-driven existence will make life meaningful and give us long-lasting happiness.

Detachment from the Material World

All of us want to succeed in life. That is a natural and healthy need for meeting the requirements of sustaining our existence. But some of us fall prey to the pressure to want more than our fair share.

Money and material wealth have been the driving force of mankind for a very long time. The truth is, however, you cannot take these material possessions beyond the grave. Is it really worth while to kill yourself for these possessions?

Look around. All that you see is finite. It will not last forever. Humans, animals, and plants cannot exist indefinitely. Like the moon's reflection on the water, it is all an illusion. According to Buddhism, attachment is an illusion that causes suffering, while detachment leads you out of suffering. When operating with an emphasis on attachment and the accumulation of vast material wealth you are always in a state of anxiety and fear. If you do not have something, you want to get it, and if you get that desired object, you worry about losing it; and you are going to lose or spend it sooner or later. So, why bother to be so attached?

This does not mean that money is not important. We all need money to cover our basic necessities and to get what we need to keep us comfortable. Beyond that, however, we really do not need a lot. We need to learn skills to support ourselves, to work hard and have a money-saving and management plan.

If you are strapped due to lack of money to cover your basic needs of living, do an honest assessment. See that as an opportunity to improve your money management skills or to develop other abilities that provide greater financial reward. If that means furthering your education, apply yourself to such a task, no matter what your age. This effort will help you advance in professional opportunities that provide a higher standard of living.

Living In the Present

Oftentimes, we can be so caught up in our daily vicissitudes that we miss out on life's pleasurable moments. Here are 2 stories to illustrate what I mean:

> *A man fell from a cliff. He caught hold of a tree branch halfway down the cliff and was just hanging there. Looking down, he saw a group of lions lying at the base of the cliff. The branch was going to break any second, and surely he would die. At that moment, he saw a beautiful plant nearby that was bearing a gorgeous red strawberry. He plucked the strawberry, put it into his mouth and savored its delicate flavor. He felt wonderful at that very moment.*

A king posed 3 questions to the wise men in his country to help him make right decisions:

1. *What is the best time to do each thing?*
2. *Who are the most important people to work with?*
3. *What is the most important thing to do at all times?*

His answers came, and much to his surprise, they were:

1. *The most important time is now.*
2. *The most important person is the one you are with.*
3. *The most important thing to do is to make the person next to you happy.*

Yesterday is history, tomorrow is mystery, and we only have today, the present.

If we live in regret, we live in the past. If we worry a lot, we live in the future, anticipating that something bad will happen. We need to learn from our mistakes made in the past and to plan for the future, but we only have today for actually living. If we enjoy this moment, like the man hanging on the cliff, we can make today a better yesterday—that is the beginning of real effectiveness. If we do not live in the now, in our present moment, we are not truly living and savoring our lives!

Cause and Effect

We do not often stop to think about how our actions affect our well-being. But it is a fact that for every choice we make and each action we take, there is a consequence. Here's a story to illustrate:

A man walked down the street with a large hole in the ground. Not seeing the hole, he fell into it. He cursed and screamed, but eventually managed to climb out of the hole.

The next day, he walked down that same street again and saw the hole. He pretended not to see the hole and, of course, he fell into it again. He screamed and cursed, and it again took him awhile to get out.

The next day, he walked down the street and saw the hole. This time, he walked around the hole and did not fall into it.

The following day, he chose to walk along a different street.

Looking back on my life, I can see that each time I have made a mistake I have paid the price for it. Sometimes I have learned a valuable lesson and have not made the same mistake again. But many times, I repeated the same mistake until I finally realized that I must change.

In learning this valuable lesson, I had to realize that everything in life has a cause and a result. For every unpleasant thing we are experiencing, we are a part of the cause. Do not completely blame others for your misery. Look for where you are not taking actions to decrease the quotient of displeasure.

Are you letting another person push your hot buttons? Are you putting off taking an action that you have known you need to take? Are you allowing yourself to remain in a situation that causes you more harm than good? Do you need an attitude adjustment? Be realistic in such an assessment. The most important thing you can do is to know yourself so that you can respond to challenges that crop up in daily life.

If you want to harvest a certain fruit, you must first plant the seeds. If you want something to happen tomorrow, plan for it today. If you want to have a good relationship with your spouse and friends, sharpen your communication skills. If you want to find a good job, get the necessary skills through quality education and training. If you want to be financially secure, plan to save money and pay off debt.

The results you see today are from the causes you did or did not plant in the past. If you plant the cause today, you will see the result in the future. Take responsibility for your life; and remember, God helps those who help themselves.

Happiness versus Pleasure

We all want to be happy, and we all want to have pleasure. Is happiness equal to pleasure?

I once had a conversation with a patient who told me he had a successful business in the past. As CEO of the company, he had worked very hard for many years. He had sold his business at a huge profit several years ago. Since that time, he had traveled a lot, built a big house, bought fancy cars and even remarried. In the beginning, he was very happy. There were many pleasures in his life; but gradually he became bored. He felt he was not challenged intellectually, and he had too much time on his hands. Playing golf, eating gourmet food and traveling to exotic places no longer made him happy. He gained weight, began to have fights with his new wife and became depressed. He was someone who had achieved great success, but had failed at fostering his happiness.

Happiness is a state of mind that can be trained and cultivated. You do not have to be rich or pretty or have a good spouse to be happy. Happiness is a choice and a decision.

In *The Art of Happiness*, author Howard Cutler, M.D., has a conversation with the Dalai Lama, who says that the first step in seeking happiness is learning. Learn that negative emotions such as anger and hatred are not only bad and harmful to you personally but harmful to society and the future of the whole world. Once we realize that, we become determined to develop and cultivate positive emotions such as kindness, compassion and love.

To cultivate positive emotions, you first need to reduce negative emotions. Your thoughts impact your emotions. Indeed, negative thoughts foster negative emotions. It is very important, therefore, to think positively. You can see your glass as half full or half empty. That depends on what you perceive and your attitude in response to your perception. Try to find the good in everything and each person. Catch yourself before you fall into the negative thoughts and emotions that drag you down or sabotage you.

At such a time, do something to create happiness for someone else. Sometimes, just reaching out to be helpful to another person in need will make your own problems and difficulties much more miniscule. Isolation often kills the seeds of happiness. Being with others and sharing joyful moments can be so rewarding. Or confiding in someone you deeply trust can cut your burden in half so that you can better enjoy what the moment has to offer.

There are many ways to foster happiness. Pursue those means, make them a high priority in your life, and your resultant good cheer will be an inspiration for others.

Pain and Suffering

A friend once asked me: "If God is so mighty and loving, why is there so much suffering in the world?"

There are different types of suffering. One is self-inflicted from shame, fear, anxiety, depression, or hatred. We can reduce this type of suffering by learning how to release these negative emotions. If you find it difficult to do this on your own, a professional counselor can help you do that quite effectively.

Other forms of suffering are a normal part of human life, such as getting old and sick or facing death. We all go through this process and, hopefully, we can value and appreciate life all the more when we are sensitively in touch with our mortality.

In the Old Testament, Joseph was sold by his brothers as a slave and taken to Egypt. He was later imprisoned due to a wrongful accusation, but Joseph never complained. Later on, when he was advisor to the pharaoh and in charge of all Egypt, his brothers came for food during a terrible drought. At this time, he revealed himself to his brothers. "Do not be angry with yourselves," he said; "God sent me here ahead of you to preserve your lives."

This is a great example of forgiveness and finding the purpose of life through pain and suffering.

A Chinese proverb says: "Before heaven gives a man big responsibilities, he must pass the test of suffering of the mind and body." I have seen people who have had an easy life, yet they have never achieved anything. Conversely, many great people have had humble and even harsh beginnings to their lives, but have gone on to achieve great things.

Perhaps pain and suffering is God's training ground for developing stronger spiritual muscles so that we can take on more responsibilities later. It is helpful to remember that we are never alone in our suffering. Staying close to those in our support system at such a time can be quite sustaining when difficulties arise.

Always remember: "There are no royal roads, shortcuts or easy paths to Paradise." The suffering that is ours today is not very different from the pain that others experience in the course of their lives. What is more, our suffering helps us develop sensitivity to the pain that others must bear. Indeed, much compassion results from the great tragedies we experience in life, and that makes us more useful to helping others in times of difficulty.

Forgiveness Toward Ourselves and Others

When Jesus was crucified, he said on the cross regarding his executioners: "Father, forgive them for they know not what they do."

There is no greater forgiveness than this. Forgiveness is the way that leads to love. If we do not forgive, we cannot love. Our spouses are the best people on which to practice forgiveness. Indeed, if you do not forgive, it is like you are drinking poison with the futile hope that your enemy will die. If you do not forgive, you will never have a happy marriage or a loving relationship.

Humans make mistakes, sometimes on purpose and oftentimes by accident. When a mistake occurs, the damage done is physical or emotional, or both. In fact, words can do more damage than knives sometimes, so choose your words wisely.

It is important to forgive ourselves and others. When you cannot find it within you to forgive yourself, you will ultimately feel guilty and depressed. The healthier approach is to view the mistake you have made as an opportunity to learn and to make sure not to repeat the same mistake. Apologize sincerely if you have hurt another, not just to escape the consequences. Try to make it up to the other party.

As to forgiving others, remember we are all from one source—God. If God forgives us for our errors, how can we not forgive the errors of others? Plus, if we do not forgive others, we continue to fill ourselves with anger, hatred, and resentment. These negative emotions will destroy our happiness, so we will ultimately pay the price for the mistakes made by others. Only through forgiveness can we let go of the pain. Then we can move on and heal our wounds.

Acceptance

We often prefer to look the other way when we stubbornly cling to something that no longer serves us well. Our rigid patterns can be a major source of our suffering and sorrow.

Then there are times when things just do not seem to go our way. We have been diligent and worked hard for important goals, but we may be thwarted by seemingly insurmountable obstacles. Or perhaps someone else is a source of profound difficulty, and nothing we do helps to improve that troubled relationship.

Knowing what to do better in those circumstances is difficult at best. This is when the principle of acceptance comes into play. The Serenity Prayer by Reinhold Niebuhr is helpful in such a situation:

God, give us grace to accept with serenity
the things that cannot be changed,
Courage to change the things
which should be changed,
and the Wisdom to distinguish
the one from the other.

Living one day at a time;
Enjoying one moment at a time;
Accepting hardship as a pathway to peace;
Taking, as Jesus did, this sinful world
as it is, not as I would have it;
Trusting that You will make all things right,
if I surrender to Your will;
So that I may be reasonably happy in this life,
and supremely happy with You
Forever in the next.
Amen

Having exhausted all possibilities of action for bettering our life situation, then it is time to accept where we are and make the most of it. Gradually, change will occur. Nothing stays static forever; but while waiting for the shift, it is wise to accept the present moment and be at peace with it. From this serene awareness arises the ability to make positive changes as opportunities appear.

Love

We hear about love all the time. Love has been praised in different cultures through different ages. We all want to love and be loved. But what is love?

I once spoke to a young man about his family. He told me he had been married for a few years and had two young children. He loved his wife and children, but he also felt that his wife complained too much. So, he was contemplating a divorce. I asked what his wife complained about. He said: "I work long hours and, when I get done with work, I do not want to be bothered with my children. When I have time during the weekend, I like to play ball with my friends and hang out in a bar. My wife complains that I do not spend enough time with her and the children, and she is very unhappy. But if I do what she wants, I feel deprived and unhappy. I have thought about divorce because I can have my freedom again and there are plenty of women still interested in me."

I replied: "I think what you mean is that you still love your wife because you want to have sex with her. You love your children as long as they do not bother you. Do you call this love? If you really love your children, you need to spend time with them even when you are tired. You need to provide a secure environment for them as they grow up. If you love your wife, you need to find out what bothers her and seek better communications, and look for solutions to the problems so that you both can accept."

Love is action. Love is doing good things for people with their best interests at heart. Love is seeing what other people need before they even think to ask for help. Love is kind words and constructive suggestions, not criticism. Love requires a lot of work and is not always pleasant. Loving others sometimes requires self-sacrifice.

Romantic love is the most fragile type of love. Oftentimes it is lust with a generous helping of our own illusions. Once reality hits, romantic love can evaporate like the morning fog.

Paul said it quite well in the New Testament (II Corinthians 13:4-7):

Love is patient and kind.
Love is not jealous or boasting or proud or rude.
Love does not demand its own way.
Love is not irritable, and it keeps no record of when it has been wronged.
It is never glad about injustice, but rejoices whenever truth wins out.
Love never gives up, never loses faith, is always hopeful, and endures through every circumstance.

Duality versus Oneness

One of my all time favorite movies is Star Wars. It fascinated me to see the character of Darth Vader, who began life as a smart young boy and was trained as a Jedi master; but because of the fear and greed in him, he eventually turned to the dark side. At the end of his life, he died for his son, the young Skywalker, and become a good person again as he showed his love.

Good and evil, happiness and sadness, love and hate—these things seem so opposite, yet both exist together. They are just different sides of the same thing. If we separate ourselves from God, we have more the dark side. If we are with God, we have more the good side. It is our choice.

We need to see the oneness in everybody and everything, because we are all from God. When we can see that and act upon that, there will be no more hatred and violence. We will develop love and compassion toward everything.

Connecting to Our Higher Power with Prayer and Meditation

I believe that when God created us, He invested His spirit in us. I view His spirit as our higher mind, the God within us. When you draw a cup of water from the ocean, the structure of the water in the cup is the same as in the ocean. Separated from its source, the water in the cup will dry out, evaporate. If we separate from our creator, we will not be happy.

There are ways to stay connected to God, however. Both prayer and meditation are effective techniques for maintaining this life-giving connection. When we pray, we ask for guidance and wisdom, we ask for help and forgiveness and we give God our thanks and appreciation for all that we have. When we are able to express gratitude even for our difficulties, we are empowered to meet those challenges more creatively and dynamically. We are emboldened to develop along spiritual lines, even as we grow in our human abilities.

It is only through awareness of what God and other people have done for us that we can appreciate what we have. Rather than being proud that we are better than other people or depressed that we do not have enough of certain things, we can instead be truly humble and content with all that we do have. We can aspire to better our situation in life through consistent application of our bountiful intelligence and creative solutions to overcoming obstacles.

If prayer is sending our message to God, then meditation is the act of providing receptivity for the answer. When you quiet your busy mind, then ideas may come forth spontaneously. This is how creativity and plans of action begin.

Prayer for the self, such as finding a good job or getting over a disease, are good but are a lower form of prayer. Prayer for other people's well being and meditating to perceive God's guidance is a higher form of prayer and worship, as it demonstrates sincere appreciation for God's indwelling spirit, that inspires us to excel at our utmost.

Religion versus Spirituality

Not everybody agrees there is a particular God, but almost everybody agrees that there is an intelligent force that moves the universe. The word "spiritual" originated from the Latin word "breathing." We need to breathe to live. Spirituality makes our life meaningful.

A religion is a collection of beliefs, which leads us to see the world in a certain way, and causes us to become more spiritual though religious practice. Like all roads that lead to Rome, all religions should lead us to spirituality; some, however, may take more time than others. If a religion makes us feel filled with guilt and shame, it is not a good religion. If a religion makes us become hateful and violent, it is not a true religion.

Spirituality can also be achieved though nonreligious pathways as long as we are compassionate and attuned to the principles we discussed above.

Years ago I went to Indonesia and visited Bora Badu, an ancient Buddhist monument and meditation tower. Carved on the stonewall of the first level, are the pictures of human suffering—being born, getting old, becoming sick and dying. On the second level, people are more spiritual and thus there is less suffering. On the third level, human beings become Buddha, enlightened, and formless.

An enlightened or spiritually advanced person is someone who achieves great peace and joy after working through the issues and problems of their lives. An enlightened person is someone who is awakened spiritually, redirecting their energy to higher traits and thus living a more purposeful life. An enlightened person walks with God all the time.

We are all on different levels of spiritual pathways. If we cultivate inner happiness, exhibit kindness and compassion towards one another and follow the principles that lead to a peaceful and truly meaningful existence we will be helping the world and ourselves so that someday we can all be enlightened.

Part IV:

Healthy Aging Program

CHAPTER 16

Prevention of Disease

Reaching mid-life can be a wonderful time in our lives, one filled with happiness, prosperity, and a deep sense of fulfillment. Thanks to integrated approaches like pellet therapy that help us to balance the vital aspects of our health needs, we know that reaching middle-age does not have to herald a decline in our health and well being. Physically, we can be as vital as ever, affording the time and energy we need to look back, treasure the lessons we have learned and share our experiences with others in anticipation of many happy and vital years to come.

While it is true that mid-life is a time when our bodies become more susceptible to chronic and debilitating diseases, there are a remarkable number of preventative measures you can take to dramatically improve and maintain your health, as well as forestall most debilitating diseases. The key to prevention is awareness. This chapter examines some of the most pressing diseases that pose particular risks to those in the mid-life stage, as well as discusses steps that can be taken to strengthen the body's internal systems, stay healthy, and prevent the onset of disease.

Cardiovascular Disease—Hypertension, Heart Attack, and Stroke

Cardiovascular disease affects the body's heart and blood vessels. It is the number one killer of men and women worldwide. In the United States alone, it accounts for over 40 percent of all deaths, more than all forms of cancer combined.

Heart disease develops gradually over many years due to atherosclerosis, or hardening of the arteries. Healthy arteries are strong and flexible. As the walls of the arteries become thick and stiff, blood circulation is reduced. When an artery becomes totally occluded (blocked), the surrounding tissues are then blocked from their supply of oxygen and nutrients delivered by the blood vessels. As a result, the surrounding tissues die, which triggers a heart attack if the tissue is in the heart, or a stroke if the tissue is in the brain.

For many years, cholesterol has been singled out as a major culprit of hardening of the blood vessels. More and more recent evidence, however, shows that inflammation of the blood vessels also plays an important role in the cause of atherosclerosis.

A common illustration explains this point. If you cook food in a new pan with a nonstick surface, the food will not adhere to the pan. When the pan has been used a lot, the food begins to stick to the surface where it has been scratched. The same principle applies to blood vessels.

They are very smooth, and normally cholesterol will not deposit in the arterial walls. When the blood vessels become inflamed, their surface becomes roughened. This allows cholesterol, along with calcium and other materials, to attach to the arterial wall resulting in the formation of plaque. As the plaque grows on the lining of the blood vessel wall, the wall itself can rupture, leading to occlusion of the artery, causing the occurrence of a heart attack or stroke. Or, circulation can get sluggish enough that the blood cells and platelets clump together and form a clot that blocks the blood vessel.

This, too, results in either a heart attack or stroke. It also explains why many people can have a heart attack or stroke while still showing normal levels of cholesterol. The heart attack or stroke is due to the underlying inflammation of the blood vessel wall that precipitates the formation of plaque. This is why normalizing the cholesterol level does not completely prevent cardiovascular disease.

What causes inflammation of the blood vessels? While there is much about inflammation that is not yet known, the causes for inflammation in the blood vessels that we do know about are free radicals, oxidative stress from lack of antioxidants due to inadequate nutrition, or exposure to environmental hazards such as smoking, toxins and heavy metals. Inflammation is a condition to be avoided as much as possible, as it also is a significant causative factor of cancer, arthritis, autoimmune diseases, Alzheimer's disease, and premature aging, to name a few.

We know inflammation devours nitric oxide, which leads to constriction of the blood vessels. Stress hormones, such as epinephrine (adrenaline) and norepinephrine, also constrict blood vessels. Constriction of blood vessel walls leads to an increase in blood pressure; the increased pressure on the blood vessels also contributes to inflammation. It becomes a vicious cycle. This is the physiology of how long-term stress, environmental toxins, and nutritional deficiency, along with other factors such as lack of exercise, obesity, smoking, and diabetes lead to hypertension and cardiovascular disease.

Diagnostic Tests for Screening Cardiovascular Diseases

1. Lipid panel

The lipid panel includes triglycerides, high-density lipoproteins (HDL, or good cholesterol), and low-density lipoproteins (LDL, or bad cholesterol), total cholesterol, and HDL/LDL ratio. More advanced testing will include small, dense LDL; and Lp(a)(very dense LDL). Both are smaller than the larger buoyant LDL and can enter blood vessels easier, and cause atherosclerosis.

2. CRP (C-reactive protein)

CRP (C-reactive protein) is an inflammation indicator. Hs-CRP (highly sensitive CRP) is a more specific indicator for blood vessel inflammation.[69,70]

3. Homocysteine

Many studies link an increased homocysteine level with the risk of heart attack and stroke.[71] Homocysteine damages the blood vessel wall and leads to inflammation. Elevated homocysteine is usually due to inadequate detoxification. It can be reduced in two ways. The first is methylation, a major process in phase II liver detoxification pathway. This occurs when methyl groups are assimilated by homocysteine and it becomes methionine (an amino acid), and S-adenosyl methionine (SAMe). This process requires the vitamin folic acid and vitamin B12. The second is a process called transsulfuration, where homocysteine is converted to cysteine. This process requires vitamin B6. I interpret a higher homocysteine level as meaning that the body needs more help in the detoxifying process. A normal homocysteine level is below 15 μmol/L, while an optimal level is under 7 μmol/L. Take vitamins B6, B12 and folic acid if your homocysteine level is not in the optimal range.

4. Fibrinogen

Fibrinogen is a protein involved in the formation of blood clots. A higher fibrinogen level leads to increased platelet aggregation and hypercoagulation. This can be dangerous, especially if the blood vessel linings are inflamed. The inflammation attracts platelets and fibrinogen to form blood clots that block the arteries, often with disastrous results. Many people take a blood thinner such as aspirin to prevent the platelet aggregation that leads to heart attacks and strokes. Natural sources for platelet aggregation inhibitors are vitamin E, green tea, garlic, and ginkgo biloba.

5. Insulin, Blood Sugar, and HbA1c

By illustration, when you make dough for home-baked bread it is very soft, but becomes hard as it is baked. Just as baking bread hardens the soft dough, a higher blood sugar level creates changes in protein structures. Hemoglobin (Hb) is a protein that changes into HbA1c in proportion to higher blood sugar levels. Thus it is a standard test to screen for diabetes and to follow in patients with diabetes. The normal range for HbA1c is under 6%; below 5.2% is optimal. Higher sugar intake triggers increased insulin production from the pancreas to handle the elevated sugar load. The protein conversion and higher insulin level ultimately leads to atherosclerosis, heart attacks and strokes, which happens in many patients with diabetes.

6. Body Scan

This radiology test screens for calcification of blood vessels in the body. It is not 100 percent accurate because if the plaque is not calcified, it will not show up in the scan. However, it can screen for atherosclerosis at an early stage. Other tests, such as the treadmill, echocardiogram, or Cardiolite nuclear testing, are not able to pick up early stages of atherosclerosis.

Prevention of Cardiovascular Disease

There are many proactive steps you can take today to reduce your risk of cardiovascular disease.

1. Diet

Eating a nutritious, balanced diet that is high in fruits and vegetables helps to reduce inflammation, cholesterol, and homocysteine. For details see the anti-inflammation diet in chapter 9.

2. Exercise

Regular exercise is essential to good health. It helps reduce blood pressure by dilating blood vessels, increasing endorphins; improving muscle tone; strengthening the heart, lungs and bones; lowering cholesterol; and reducing weight. Furthermore, exercise helps the body to detoxify by improving blood circulation and lymphatic drainage. Vigorous exercise also stimulates the secretion of growth hormone, which has many beneficial effects upon the body. Yoga and Qigong are relaxing exercises that reduce blood pressure effectively.

3. Stress Reduction

Positive thinking, meditating, deep breathing, getting adequate sleep, managing time wisely, building good relationships, controlling anger, and finding a purpose for your life are all important to reduce stress, and to better adjust to stressful situations. This also helps to keep your hormones and body chemicals in proper balance.

4. Balance Your Hormones

Testosterone for men and estrogen for women are known to improve cardiovascular health. High cortisol, adrenaline, and high insulin levels lead to high blood pressure and inflammation of blood vessel walls. Check your hormone levels and treat hormone deficiency adequately.

5. Supplements

Recommended daily doses of supplements include:

- Magnesium citrate, 400-800 mg; and potassium, 500-800 mg, which help blood vessel dilation and reduce blood pressure.[72]

- Co-Q10, 100-300 mg; and L-carnitine, 100-200 mg, which improve mitochondria energy production and heart function.

- Arginine, 3,000 mg, stimulates the production of the potent vasodilator nitrous oxide as well as the secretion of growth hormone.

- Folic acid (folate), 800 mcg; vitamin B6, 100 mg; and vitamin B12, 400 mcg, which help to lower homocysteine and assist in the detoxification process.

- Vitamin C, 1,000 mg; vitamin E, 400-800 IU; selenium, 100 mg; and beta-carotene, 25,000 IU, which are all antioxidants that neutralize free radicals.

- Omega-3 fatty acids, 1,500 mg, are important in reducing inflammation of the blood vessels.

— Fiber, such as grounded flaxseed fiber 1-2 tablespoons with each meal helps to reduce fat and sugar absorption. It also helps with cholesterol excretion.

Cancer

The big "C" is a terrifying word. It is the second most common cause of death in all age groups, but it is the number one cause of death in people under 70 years old.

The most common cancers are of the lung, colon, breast and prostate. In 1970 President Nixon declared war on cancer, expecting to find a cure by 1990. Unfortunately, the rate of cancer has increased instead, especially the hormone-dependent cancers such as breast and prostate cancer.

Cancer is often due, among other factors, to DNA mutation. What causes this mutation? Inflammation, particularly resulting from exposure to environmental toxins, leads to the development of cancer.[73,74] I believe cancer is mostly due to environmental factors, such as chronic stress, smoking and toxin exposure, but genetic predisposition also plays a significant role, probably through inadequate detoxification enzymes.

Diagnostic Testing for Early Cancer Detection

There are several approaches to screening for cancer; including history and physical exam, blood tests, radiological tests, and additional tests.

- **History and Physical Exam**

Physicians will take a medical history of the patient and conduct a physical exam, which includes:

— Examining the thyroid nodule and lymph nodes.

— A digital rectal exam for rectal and prostate cancer.

— Breast palpation for unusual lumps.

- A skin inspection for pigmented lesions, moles or ulcerations that do not heal.

- **Blood Tests**

  - The only blood test that is good for cancer screening is the PSA (prostate specific antigen) for prostate cancer. It is recommended once a year for men over 50 years old.

  - CEA for colon cancer and CA 125 for ovarian cancer, but these are not good for screening, primarily because these indicators do not show up until the later stages of cancer. Also, these indicators can increase due to benign conditions making them nonspecific, which creates the need to rule out other causes. The best use of these two tests is to monitor for recurrence of cancer after treatment.

- **Radiological Tests**

  There are several radiological tests that can be utilized to help detect certain forms of cancer.

  - Mammograms. The mammogram for breast cancer screening is still standard and needs to be done once a year for women over 50 years old. Unfortunately, the mammogram is not accurate when breast tissues are dense, thus it is not a good screening tool for women younger than 40 years old. The newer digital mammogram is better in terms of clarity.

    The breast MRI (magnetic resonance imaging) is also available now, but its use is limited due to cost. A breast ultrasound is usually done after the mammogram if there is an area with increased density. If questions persist, then the MRI is used for greater diagnostic resolution.

    Thermogram of the breast, which uses infrared imaging, has been around for awhile but is not considered standard screening. The theory behind thermography is that if cancer cells are growing in a certain area, the blood supply and temperature of that location will increase. This makes it good for early detection, but it can be nonspecific due to other conditions, such as infection.

Most importantly, women of all ages should learn how to do breast exams and do them regularly. I have seen patients who had a negative mammogram but had a palpable lump that a biopsy identified as cancer. If there is a strong family history of breast cancer, genetic testing for BRCA 1 and BRCA 2 may be valuable, too.

— Chest X-ray. A chest X-ray for lung cancer screening is recommended once a year for those over 50 years old, as well as for high-risk groups, chiefly smokers. CT (computer tomography) of the chest is more accurate, but its use is limited due to cost and radiation exposure. It is often used if the screening chest X-ray shows an abnormality suspicious for cancer.

— Colonoscopy. A lower GI (barium enema) or colonoscopy is done to screen for colon cancer. The preparation for both procedures is the same. The colonoscopy is more expensive and more invasive. It is recommended for high-risk populations, such as those with a family history of colon cancer, chronic inflammation of the bowel such as ulcerative colitis, Crohn's disease, irritable bowel syndrome, or chronic constipation. Generally, it is done once every ten years for people over 50 years old. This is frequent enough, unless a polyp (growth) is discovered; then a colonoscopy needs to be done every three to five years, with biopsies of any polyps for possible cancer.

— Endoscope. Endoscope is routinely performed in Japan as a screening test for stomach cancer because the Japanese have a high rate of stomach cancer. It is not routinely done in the U.S., but it is probably a good idea for people who have stomach problems, especially among the Asian population. Another very common cancer among Asians is liver cancer associated with chronic hepatitis B. For them, an abdominal ultrasound is recommended yearly.

— Body scan. A body scan is a better tool for early detection of cancer and heart diseases. However, it is not 100 percent accurate and can have many false positives, which can lead to unnecessary procedures having to be performed. For those over 50 years old, I do recommend that it be done about every ten years.

- **Other Tests**

Additional tests include Pap cytology for cervical cancer, and urinalysis for blood in the urine, which can be due to kidney or bladder cancer. Sputum cytology for lung cancer, if there is chronic productive cough; stool guaiac occult blood for colon cancer; and biopsies for suspicious lumps or skin lesions that do not heal.

Cancer Prevention

There are many simple, yet powerful steps you can take to minimize your risk of cancer.

1. **Avoid Cancer-causing (Carcinogenic) Sources**

— Do not smoke, and avoid secondhand smoke.

— Avoid xenohormones or hormone disruptors, such as meat from animals injected with hormones, as well as pesticides, bug killers, and plastics.

— Avoid processed foods that contain artificial food colors, sweeteners and preservatives.

— Avoid hair dyes, cosmetics, perfumes or deodorants that contain toxic chemicals.

— Avoid drinking chlorinated tap water.

— Avoid wrapping food in plastic wrap or aluminum foil.

2. Diet

A cancer-avoidance nutritional base diet should focus on toxin avoidance and detoxification and include:

— A large number of servings of organically grown vegetables, especially cruciferous ones such as broccoli, cabbage, Brussels sprouts, and cauliflower, which help the liver detoxify and provide antioxidants to neutralize free radicals.

— Citrus fruits, such as oranges, lemons, limes and tangerines, which are high in vitamin C.

— Increased fiber through vegetables or foods like ground flax seed.

— Drinking plenty of water: 50 percent of your weight in ounces (for example, 100 lbs. = 100 ounces).

— Reducing animal meats, especially those that are nitrate-cured or smoked, and high in animal fats.

— Reducing sugar and other refined carbohydrates.

3. Stress Reduction

— Be in tune with your inner child. Write down your feelings and emotions on a daily basis. Let go of the negative emotions, and cultivate the positive emotions.

— Practice meditation, deep breathing, and creative imaging. Regularly engage in relaxation exercises, such as yoga.

— Find purpose in your life. Set goals. Plan for the future, and prioritize your activities.

— Do simple things that bring you joy, such as walking on the beach, taking a relaxing bath, getting a massage, listening to your favorite music, or dancing. Do these activities regularly.

— Associate frequently with good friends who are supportive, and do fun things together.

— Laugh a lot. Laughter is often the best medicine.

4. Regular Exercise

Exercise has many overall health benefits. For cancer prevention, it improves circulation and aids in the detoxification process. Exercise also improves immunity by bringing more nutrition and oxygen to organs and tissues.

5. Hormone Balance

Many hormones, such as estrogen, progesterone, testosterone and melatonin help with sleep quality. This leads to improved immunity and an overall sense of well-being. When we are feeling good and energetic, we tend to take better care of ourselves and others, too.

6. Supplements

— Antioxidants daily dosage includes vitamin C, 1,000 mg; vitamin E, 400-800 IU; beta-carotene, 25,000 IU; and selenium, 100 mg; all of which neutralize free radicals and help the detoxification process.

— Fiber, such as ground flax seed, psyllium, or apple pectin helps the detoxification process.

— Omega-3 fatty acids, 1,500 mg to help reduce inflammation.

Metabolic Syndrome—Insulin Resistance, Obesity, and Diabetes

Metabolic syndrome entails a collection of negative health factors that lead to developing insulin resistance, fatty degeneration of the liver, heart disease, and type II diabetes. It is estimated that over 50 million people in America fit into the clinical profile of metabolic syndrome. Indeed, more than 20 million people are diagnosed with diabetes and among those, 90 percent have type II (adult onset) diabetes. The remaining 10 percent have type I (juvenile) diabetes.

In the year 2000, the U.S. spent roughly $2 billion on the treatment of diabetes. Obesity, often a factor in diabetes, reached epidemic levels at the new millennium, and most members of this group already have, or are on their way to developing metabolic syndrome, diabetes, and heart disease, unless they change their lifestyle and eating habits.

Metabolic syndrome is a constellation of obesity, elevated cholesterol and triglycerides, along with a high insulin level. Insulin is a hormone manufactured by specialized glands in the pancreas that facilitate the transportation of sugar from the bloodstream into the tissues and cells. This syndrome begins with over eating; particularly high glycemic-index carbohydrates, such as breads, pastas, potatoes, rice, or desserts. In response to an inundation of these high-glycemic foods, the body secretes insulin to handle the sugar load.

A higher sugar load translates to higher insulin demand. If the body does not burn off the sugar immediately, it stores it in a lighter form, which is fat. As a person continues to over eat sugars (carbohydrates), the body gains fat. Initially the fat goes primarily to the abdominal area, then the subcutaneous (under the skin) fat layers throughout the body, then the muscle, the whole body, and eventually to the liver. When this occurs, the condition is referred to as fatty liver.

Another factor in metabolic syndrome is insulin resistance.[75] As greater amounts of fat are stored in the cell membrane (outer covering), it becomes insensitive to insulin and the body has to secrete higher levels of insulin to handle the same sugar load. If a person continues to over eat foods loaded with high-glycemic carbohydrates, even with increased production of insulin, the body cannot handle the sugar load. The result is the beginning of an increase in the blood sugar in the blood stream, which leads to type II diabetes.

Type I diabetes results from the pancreas being destroyed by a viral infection, or an autoimmune disease, which leads to its inability to secrete insulin. This form of diabetes usually starts at a much younger age and requires treatment by insulin injections. The treatment for type II diabetes is not insulin; it is simply a reduced sugar load, although certain medications in pill form can help somewhat in controlling the high blood sugar levels.

High insulin provokes inflammation by triggering pro-inflammatory cytokines. High insulin causes a lipoprotein lipase deficiency, which leads to increased triglycerides and decreased HDL (the good cholesterol). A fatty liver also contributes to increased inflammation, since the burdened liver is not able to detoxify as well as a normal liver. Toxins can certainly cause more inflammation. Inflammation of the blood vessel walls and high cholesterol leads to atherosclerosis (hardening of the arteries) and hypertension. Hypertension, diabetes and hyperlipidemia (high cholesterol) lead to heart attacks and strokes.

Laboratory Testing

When checking for diabetes and metabolic syndrome, these are the most common tests physicians will perform.

1. Insulin Level

A normal fasting insulin level is 3 to 28; the optimal range is below 5.

2. HbA1c

HbA1c is the most important test for diabetes. As stated earlier in this chapter, the normal range for HbA1c is 4.8% to 6.0%; below 5.2% is optimal, and should be measured every three months for diabetic patients.

3. Lipid Profile

Prevention and Treatment of Metabolic Syndrome

There are many things you can do to prevent and treat metabolic syndrome, starting with a diet to lose weight.

1. Weight loss diet. Please see pages 133-134 for details.

2. Supplements. It is very important to take supplements if you have metabolic syndrome in order to reduce inflammation, improve insulin sensitivity, lower cholesterol, and improve detoxification.

   — Fiber slows down the absorption of glucose, increases the excretion of cholesterol, decreases constipation, and provides a feeling of fullness, which helps to reduce the appetite and thereby lose weight. However, water-soluble fiber is fermented by intestinal bacteria and can cause gas, so it is better to start slowly. Fiber also needs to be taken with plenty of water. I recommend psyllium seed, ground flax seed, or Benefiber. Take 1 tablespoon in a large glass of water or tea and drink it before or with meals.

   — High-potency multiple vitamins and minerals provide a base of antioxidants and important vitamins and minerals, such as chromium, magnesium, vanadium, zinc, selenium, vitamins C, E, and B complex. These neutralize free radicals and promote better function of insulin.

   — Omega-3 fish oil reduces inflammation. Use pharmaceutical grade to avoid heavy metals and environmental toxins. Buy fish oil that is free of mercury, cadmium, lead, PCBs, and other contaminants.

   — Herbs that can improve insulin functions and sensitivities, such as gymnema sylvestre, American and Korean ginseng, and fenugreek.

— Coenzyme Q10, L-carnitine, and alpha lipoic acid, which help with energy production and weight loss.

3. Exercise is absolutely an essential part of recovery from metabolic syndrome. Exercise directly improves insulin sensitivity and blood sugar. Other benefits are that it increases muscle mass and helps to burn off fat; it lowers total cholesterol and raises HDL (the good cholesterol); it burns off calories to help lose weight; and it reduces blood pressure.

4. Stress reduction and lifestyle change. Do not smoke, as smoking generates a plethora of free radicals that damage the body. Do not drink alcohol, as it exacerbates a fatty liver. Stress increases cortisol, which leads to increased blood sugar and insulin. Stress also increases adrenaline, which elevates blood pressure.

5. Balance your hormones. Normal levels of testosterone and estrogen improve insulin sensitivity and function, which lead to healthy blood sugar levels. Adequate thyroid hormone levels are needed for energy production and weight loss. Get your hormones checked if you are overweight and have high blood pressure or high blood sugar.

6. Reduce exposure to environmental toxins and take detoxification supplements, since a fatty liver impairs the ability of the liver to detoxify properly. An accumulation of toxins leads to more inflammation, sluggish metabolism and weight gain.

Premature Brain Aging, Memory Loss, Neurodegenerative Disease, Impaired Cognition, and Dementia

Most parts of the body go through constant renewal. Skin cells regenerate each month, for instance, while red blood cells regenerate every four months. But we die with the same brain cells with which we were born. They do not regenerate. Once they are gone, they are gone forever. That is why head injuries, toxins accumulating in brain cells, or impaired circulation of oxygen and nutrients to the brain cause inflammation and neurodegenerative diseases, which manifest in a variety of ways from memory loss to Alzheimer's disease.

Causes of Premature Brain Aging

It is frightening to think that the brain can die before the rest of the body, yet this is what occurs with dementia and other brain disorders. Here are contributors to this horrific condition:

- Chronic inflammation caused by toxins and free radicals.
- Nutritional deficiencies resulting from improper diet.
- Decreased oxygen and nutrients delivered to brain cells due to impaired circulation as a result of atherosclerosis, stroke or heart attack.
- Hormone deficiencies, especially testosterone, estrogen, and thyroid hormone.
- Poor lifestyle habits, such as smoking, excessive consumption of alcohol, street drugs, stress, and lack of exercise.

Prevention of Neurodegenerative Diseases

The consequences of brain cell loss can be catastrophic, but there are simple steps you can take right now to protect the health of your brain cells and minimize the risk of neurodegenerative diseases.

1. Commit to a healthy-aging diet geared toward reducing inflammation as outlined in chapter 9. Pay particular attention to:

   — Consuming lots of antioxidants from eating fresh organic fruits and vegetables of all colors.

   — Avoiding processed foods and bad fats.

— Foods rich in omega-3 fatty acids, especially DHA (docosahexaenoic acid), which is essential as the building blocks of the brain cell membranes.

— Eating good proteins as a source of amino acids that turn into neurotransmitters.

2. Avoid brain injuries. Wear protective headgear when riding a bike and participating in impact-sports.

3. Avoid using alcohol, tobacco, recreational drugs or unnecessary prescription drugs.

4. Avoid toxins as much as possible and detoxify as needed.

5. Make exercise a priority, especially aerobic exercise, which delivers more nutrients and oxygen to the brain cells. Exercise increases brain endorphins, nature's antidepressants. Deep breathing and relaxation exercises help relax the body and also increase the supply of oxygen to brain cells.

6. Exercise your brain.

   — Learn new skills such as dancing or playing the piano.

   — Engage in creative writing.

   — Play chess or solve puzzles.

   — Use your senses (touch, smell, vision and hearing) to stimulate brain functions by engaging in aromatherapy, music therapy, sculpture, or reading.

   — Engage in social interactions. Meaningful conversation can improve thought processes.

7. Stress reduction. High cortisol levels impair brain functions. Positive thoughts, joyful moments, and laughter help the neuroendocrine system to work optimally.

8. Prevent diseases such as obesity, hypertension, cardiovascular disease and diabetes, which decrease the blood supply to the brain and impair its function.

9. Balance hormones. Replace hormone deficiencies; especially testosterone, estrogen, thyroid, melatonin, DHEA, and growth hormone.

10. Use nutritional supplements.

    — Omega-3 fatty acids in fish oil. Fish has long been referred to as brain food because the basic building blocks of brain cells are EPA (eicosapentaenoic acid) and DHA (docosahexaenoic acid), which are both derived from fish oil. These fatty acids also reduce inflammation, and thus help prevent premature brain aging.

    — High-potency antioxidants and minerals.

    — Co-Q10, alpha lipoic acid and acetyl-L carnitine. All of these nutrients are needed in the mitochondria, which are the energy furnaces of the cell. Co-Q10, a coenzyme, is in all of the body's cells, particularly the heart and brain cells. These supplements help prevent brain aging by several different mechanisms, such as reducing free radicals and enhancing cellular energy and functions.

    — Choline, an essential nutrient usually grouped with the vitamin B complex, and lecithin are the precursors to acetylcholine, the neurotransmitter involved in memory.

    — Phosphatidylserine (PS) plays an important role in maintaining the brain cell membrane. By protecting the brain cell membrane, PS facilitates the transportation of nutrients into brain cells.

    — Herbs such as ginkgo biloba and vinpocetine improve circulation to the brain.

In today's world, people are living healthier and longer lives than ever before. As we age, it becomes much more essential to keep our body and mind fit in order to experience optimal energy, clarity, and balance in our day-to-day lives. Although reaching the mid-life stage can make us more susceptible to debilitating diseases, it is important to remember that taking simple steps to improve our well being each day can make us stronger, healthier and far more resistant to aging and diseases than ever before.

Following the steps outlined in this chapter will go a long way towards preserving your life-long health.

CHAPTER 17

8 Weeks to Vitality

Do you want to experience more energy each day? Do you want a clear, focused mind; an even, balanced mood; and a zest for life you have not known in years? It is within your reach. One of the most common questions I get from my patients is how to integrate all of the information I give them on improving their health into a workable, sustainable and successful program that meets their individual needs. In this chapter we are going to bring this experience to you by reviewing the entire program I use in my practice to help people achieve peak health and vitality.

Week 1
Health Assessment

1. Questionnaire for Health Assessment

Answer each question based on the following symptoms:

Point scale:

- **0** = never or almost never happens
- **1** = occasionally happens, the degree is not severe
- **2** = occasionally happens, the degree is severe
- **3** = frequently happens, the degree is not severe
- **4** = frequently happens, the degree is severe

Head

_____ Headache
_____ Dizziness
_____ Hearing loss

Eyes

_____ Watery
_____ Itching
_____ Blurred vision

Ears

_____ Ringing in ears
_____ Hearing loss
_____ Earache or infection

Nose

_____ Sneezing
_____ Congestion
_____ Postnasal drip

Mouth

_____ Sore throat
_____ Hoarseness
_____ Gum infection
_____ Toothache
_____ Canker sores
_____ Discolored tongue

Skin

_____ Acne
_____ Hives
_____ Rash
_____ Dry skin
_____ Hair loss
_____ Hot flashes

Heart

_____ Palitations or irregular heartbeat
_____ Chest pain
_____ Shortness of breath on exertion
_____ Leg edema (swelling)

Lungs

_____ Cough
_____ Asthma attack
_____ Shortness of breath

Digestive tract

_____ Nausea/vomiting
_____ Diarrhea

_____ Constipation
_____ Bloating or gas
_____ Heartburn
_____ Abdominal pain

Joints/Muscles
_____ Joint pain or stiffness
_____ Muscle pain/body ache
_____ Neck pain
_____ Back pain

Weight
_____ Weight gain
_____ Weight loss
_____ Craving certain foods
_____ Binge eating/drinking
_____ Difficulty losing weight

Energy
_____ Easily fatigued
_____ Difficulty getting up
_____ Lethargy, difficulty functioning
_____ Cold intolerance
_____ Cold hands and feet
_____ Restless/hyperactive

Sleep
_____ Difficulty falling asleep
_____ Restless sleep
_____ Frequent nightmares
_____ Wake up frequently
_____ Sleep too much

Emotions
_____ Mood swings, moodiness
_____ Anxiety, nervousness
_____ Anger/irritability
_____ Depression/loss of interest

Brain

_____ Poor memory
_____ Mental fog
_____ Difficulty concentrating
_____ Difficulty learning
_____ Confusion
_____ Headache

Immune system

_____ Frequent illness
_____ Autoimmune disease
_____ Allergies/hay fever

Gyn/Urinary tract

_____ Frequent urination
_____ Nocturia (excessive urination at night)
_____ Incontinence
_____ Urinary tract infection
_____ Genital itching or discharge
_____ Vaginal dryness or painful intercourse

[ ] **Total Score**

Results Analysis

If your score is under 5, your general health is pretty good. Between 5 and 50, it is time to take a proactive stand toward making changes that will enhance your body's health. If you have a score above 50, you are heading toward, or facing major medical issues. This also means that you need to seek medical evaluation and treatment.

This self-assessment can also be repeated over time to determine if you are moving upward or downward. If the score is coming down, you are improving. If the score is increasing, you are edging closer to health problems.

2. Laboratory Assessment

One of the first steps in helping to determine your current state of health is to run some general and specific tests.

- **General:**
  - — Blood tests, including CBC, liver and kidney functions, lipid panel, and urinalysis.
- **Specific:**
  - — Fasting insulin, HbAIc: screen for diabetes and metabolic syndrome.
  - — Homocysteine, fibrinogen, hs-CRP: screen for cardiovascular risk factors.
  - — Hormone panels: screen for thyroid, adrenal and sex hormones.

Week 2
Hormone Balance

This week is the first consultation physical examination and hormone evaluation treatment.

Hormone balance starts with bio-identical hormone replacement for both men and women if the sex hormone levels are low. I also treat subclinical hypothyroidism during this visit. Adrenal function is assessed and treated as needed.

The benefits of hormones that are balanced and at youthful levels are numerous, not the least of which is enhancing the quality of life of any individual at any age. It is also a necessary step to achieve vitality.

Week 3
Make Sleep a Priority, Check Your Stress Inventory, and Take Control

Part I. Make Sleep a Priority

With the help of hormones, you should be sleeping better now. Here are other strategies to try if you still have trouble sleeping:

1. Minimize or Avoid Stimulants

— Avoid alcohol.

— Avoid caffeine containing beverages or foods after 12 noon. This includes Pepsi, Coke, coffee or espresso, lattes, and chocolate.

— Avoid Sudafed or other over-the-counter decongestants.

— Avoid medications that may have stimulating effects.

— Avoid aerobic exercise after 6 P.M. Do relaxing exercise at night such as yoga or Pilates.

2. Avoid Nighttime Tension and Anxiety

— Avoid watching violent or anxiety provoking news, TV programs or movies at night.

— Avoid paying bills or checking the stock market before bedtime.

— Avoid arguments at night. Schedule difficult conversations at a time during the day when both parties are not emotionally disturbed. Try to achieve some resolution of the difficult issues if you have an argument before bedtime.

3. **Sleep Planning**

— Plan to sleep 8-9 hours a day and keep it the same time every day to train your biological clock. Plan to go to bed before 11 P.M. If you can go to bed around 9 to 10 P.M., it is even better.

— Avoid large meals or spicy food at least 3 hours before bed time.

— Avoid drinking liquid at least 2 hours before bedtime. Make sure you empty your bladder before going to bed so that you do not have to get up at night to go to the bathroom.

4. **Bedroom Preparation**

— Keep your bedroom air clean, especially if you have nasal congestion or are prone to snoring. Use a HEPA air filter if needed. You can use the filter for 4-6 hours before bedtime if the noise bothers you.

— Keep your bedroom quiet. Turn off any appliances or clocks that make noise. Close the window or use ear plugs if necessary.

— Decrease the light in your bedroom by turning the light off, using a window curtain, or wearing eye shades.

— Make sure the bed, pillow, and mattress are comfortable.

— Make sure the temperature in the bedroom is not too hot or too cold. Use appropriate bed covers.

— Avoid sleeping near electric fields. Try to keep your head at least 5 feet away from electric fields generated by electrical outlets, radios, clocks, computers and night lights. Avoid using an electric blanket or water bed.

5. Strategies for Falling Asleep or Staying Sleep

— Daily journal your emotions and feelings. Be in touch with your inner child. If there are things that worry you, write them down. Ask yourself how likely this is going to happen, and if this is likely to happen, ask yourself what you can do to be prepared. If this very unlikely to happen, ask yourself if you can release the unnecessary worry or fear.

— Most thoughts are recurrent thoughts. Write them down so that you do not have to think it over and over again. Meditate afterward.

— Write down the things you need to do tomorrow and prioritize them.

— Relaxation exercise such as yoga, deep breathing, and creative visualization help to unwind your busy brain waves. Use a relaxation CD or soothing music or nature sounds.

— If you still have trouble with sleep due to unsolved issues, consider counseling.

6. Supplements for Sleep

— Melatonin 0.5 mg to 2 mg sublingual before sleep.

— Magnesium citrate 400 mg to 600 mg before bedtime helps to relax the muscles and allows you to sleep deeper.

— Amino acids such as tryptophan, 5-HTP, and SAMe help to increase serotonin and GABA.

— Herbs such as valerian root or passionflower help with relaxation and sleep.

Part II. Check Your Stress Inventories and Take Control

Scientists studying the events that cause the most mental and emotional stress discovered that they have 4 characteristics in common. We are stressed by:

1. Things that are new to us.
2. Unpredictability.
3. Sense of threat.
4. Loss of control.

Life events that cause most stressful responses:

1. Death of spouse or a close family member.
2. Law suit or detention in jail.
3. Marital separation or divorce.
4. Major personal injuries or illness.
5. Major change in financial state.
6. Loss of job or being fired.
7. Changing to a different line of work, or starting new school.
8. Foreclosure on a mortgage.
9. Conflict/tension with spouse, children, in laws or other family members.
10. Major change in living conditions (moving, remodeling, etc.).

Sources of Stress

1. Work

Are you overwhelmed?

— Reorganize your work surroundings for better efficiency.

— Use an organizer to plan your day and organize tasks by priority.

Are you losing control?

— Recognize the things that you can control and forget about controlling the rest.

— If you are a control freak, get help.

Do you have difficult co workers?

— Resolve issues with supervisors and co-workers as soon as possible. Be assertive.

— Work on communication skills.

Do you hate your job?

— Find another job that you like.

— You may need more training or schooling. Make plans for a slow transition if there is financial difficulty.

2. Relationships

Relationships with our immediate family and our friends are like the fruit trees and flowers in the garden. If you planted them early and attended them regularly with love, they will bloom with beautiful flowers and yield delicious fruits. Great relationships yield great love, which is what sustains humankind. Many relationship problems are rooted in power struggles, self-centeredness, a lack of appreciation, and communication.

— Write down a list of people you enjoy being with. Make calls or arrange visits regularly so you can find joy in friendship.

— Cultivate gratitude. Being thankful and expressing your appreciation to others is therapeutic. Many times we forget to do it with those people we see everyday; our co-workers, our spouse, our children or our parents.

Remind yourself to write down daily things and people you are thankful for and make a habit to express your gratitude.

— Resolve your disputes. Relationships will eventually produce conflict. Some are minor and some are major. If left unresolved and the longer you wait, the minor ones will become major, and the major ones will become unresolvable. Make a list of people you need to resolve disputes with, and try resolving the smallest one first then move on to the next. You will find you are much less stressed, and empowered, once you have solved those conflicts.

— Forgiveness: There are times other people genuinely hurt us, physically or emotionally. Regardless of the offense, if we are unwilling to forgive, the bitterness, anger, and resentment in us will further hurt us and lead to more stress in our life. Make a list of persons you are unwilling to forgive and if you still cannot forgive them even though you tried, seek counseling with a therapist or a spiritual leader. There are times we hurt other person, consider asking forgiveness from that person and reconcile the relationship. We also need to forgive ourselves too, so the burden of guilt can be lifted.

3. Finances

Financial instability creates tremendous anxiety and stress. When an economic downturn strikes, everybody feels pinched. It is a good time to reassess our needs and wants. It is a good habit to live within our means. In the past many consumers over-extended their lifestyle; perhaps it is time to cut back and rearrange your priorities. Ask what we can learn from the situation. Remember, the most important things in life cannot be bought with money, and we do not need a lot of money to sustain our basic living.

— Down size. Simplify your life.

— Create a plan to stabilize your financial situation.

— Recognize that it might take time, but with a good plan in place, you can stop worrying.

4. Health Issues

Many health issues can be improved by simple steps:

— Taking actions to stop bad habits such as smoking or Drinking.

— Implementing good habits such as daily exercise, eating healthy meals, and taking supplements (this is your next week's home work).

— See a doctor who can help you finding the root of your illness.

Week 4
Better Nutrition and Healthy Diet

This week, start following the health aging diet that is in Chapter 9. Now is a good time to check your pantry. Throw out oils and seasonings that are over 6 months old. Get rid of cookies, candies, ice cream, cakes, diet soda, chips, and instant noodles, canned and processed foods. Buy organic virgin olive oil and cold pressed vegetable oils of your choice. Buy organic seasonings, sea salt, and raw organic nuts and seeds.

Plan your weekly meals ahead of time so that you do not have to eat on the run or eat junk fast food. Do not eat in a restaurant or take out food more than once a week. You will save a lot of money this way, money that can be used to buy organic fruits, vegetables, nuts, and seeds. Make chicken soup or bake meats during the weekend so you can use them during the week. There are a lot of delicious recipes for soups, salads, and main dishes that you can find on the internet or get from your favorite cook books.

If you are still buying bottled water or drinking from the tap, install a reverse osmosis water filter under your kitchen sink so you can get clean and filtered water.

Nutritional Supplements

Supplements help provide the body with the nutritional elements it needs for maintaining optimal performance. As a basic approach to supplementation, be sure to include high-potency antioxidants and minerals as well as mercury-free fish oils as an abundant source of omega-3 fatty acids.

For more advanced and preventive supplementation, take:

1. Digestive enzymes with each meal to aid digestion and absorption.

2. Probiotics (a source of healthy intestinal bacteria) to improve intestinal protection and function.

3. Fiber with meals to slow down absorption of sugars in food, to feed healthy intestinal bacteria, to prevent constipation and to help the detoxification process.

4. Detoxification supplements such as high dose vitamin C, amino acids, milk thistle, turmeric, broccoli extract, and alpha lipoic acid.

Week 5
Adding Exercise to Your Daily Routine

Everybody knows it is important to exercise. You may have been too tired or not motivated to exercise in the past. Now that you have more energy with the hormone treatment, it is time to make a commitment to get physically active. It takes an effective approach in order to gain its benefits.

1. Criteria for Effective Exercise

— Duration: at least 20 to 30 minutes, but not longer than an hour.

— Frequency: at least three times a week.

— Intensity: increase your heart rate to 80 percent of your target heart rate, which is 220 minus your age (220-age).

If your exercise pattern does not meet these three criteria, your body will not be able to reap the full benefits of exercise.

2. Types of Exercise

— Aerobics: such as brisk walking, jogging, playing tennis, swimming, treadmill, or bicycling. This form of exercise is beneficial for the cardiovascular system because the heart has to pump faster. It also transports more oxygen and nutrients throughout the body, especially the brain, thus preventing age-related memory loss.

— Weight training: such as lifting weights. This form of exercise helps to build muscle mass, which helps to burn body fat off, and improves body composition.

— Relaxing exercise: such as yoga, tai chi and walking. This form of exercise combines deep breathing and muscle stretching, which helps with relaxation, oxygenation and flexibility.

The best exercise is a combination of all three above. You can start by deep breathing and stretching for ten minutes, followed by jogging or any other form of aerobic exercise for 20 to 30 minutes, then deep breathing and stretching for another ten minutes as a cool down. The warm-up and cool-down phases are essential to help the muscles prepare for and recover from the exertion of exercising.

3. The Benefits of Regular Exercise

- Improves one's energy production, vitality, and sense of well-being.

- Helps the body to lose fat, builds muscle tone, and increases physical strength and endurance.

- Reduces cardiovascular diseases and improves blood circulation.

- Lowers blood pressure and cholesterol levels.

- Improves bone density and helps to prevent osteoporosis.

- Improves insulin sensitivity, reduces blood sugar, and helps to prevent diabetes and obesity.

- Improves brain function and memory, and helps to prevent senile dementia.

- Increases the level of endorphins, which helps to maintain positive moods.

- Reduces stress and stress-related diseases. Relaxes the body and mind.

- Improves the immune system, thereby reducing the incidence and severity of colds and influenzas.

- Reduces insomnia.

- Increases the body's natural production of human growth hormone, helping to reverse or slow down the aging process.

The key to making exercise a part of your lifestyle is to motivate yourself by thinking of its benefits and finding a routine that you will do regularly.

Keep a daily log of your exercise. Make it a daily routine if possible. Once it becomes a habit, it is very easy to keep. Motivate yourself by finding an exercise partner, or rewarding yourself with something you enjoy.

This week, we are also going to do another blood test to assess your hormone status, and screen for heavy metals and certain vitamins and minerals.

Week 6
Toxin Avoidance, Detoxification, and Reevaluation

Helping the body detoxify is an essential part of maintaining our health. An important first step is to avoid toxins in the environment. For toxin avoidance, please see pages 166-167; for basic detoxification, please see pages 174-175.

Check your kitchen, bathroom, laundry room, medicine cabinet, garage, and storage places. Throw away pesticides, fungicides, harsh environmental unfriendly cleaning solutions and detergents, aluminum containing deodorants and antacids, aluminum foil, aluminum canned-foods and cookware made of aluminum. Do not use plastic food wrap, thin plastic containers and Styrofoam. Check the ingredients in your cosmetics, shampoos, hair dyes and toothpaste; if you see methylparaban, benzene, sodium lauryl sulfate, chlorofluorocarbons, ammonia, or the artificial colors red/yellow/blue, it is time to replace them with products made of natural ingredients. You can usually find them in health food stores.

If you have allergies and your bedroom carpet is old and thick, change it to wood or tile. At least get a HEPA air filter if you cannot replace them right away. If your bathroom and kitchen are damp and dirty, you need to clean them well and improve the ventilation. If you have not cleaned the air ducts in your house in over 7 years, then it is time to get them cleaned.

This week is also the week of re-evaluation. Most of my patients on their return appointment report feeling a lot better already. The common issues I encounter at this stage are insufficient energy, or the inability to lose weight. This may be due to adrenal fatigue, chronic fatigue syndrome, metabolic syndrome, toxin overload, heavy metal toxicity, depression, and leaky gut or food sensitivities.

At this stage, the treatment will depend on each person's unique health issues. The modality we use at this time may include acupuncture, IV nutrition or chelation, a weight loss program, further nutritional treatments to help energy production, insulin sensitivity, healing the intestine tract, and other detoxification methods.

For those improved already, continue your healthy diet, exercise, nutritional supplements, and detoxification so you can reap more benefits.

Week 7
Unleash Your Subconscious Power

This week, we are going to work on our subconscious mind and our spirituality. We also want to put more joy in our life.

1. Set a time for meditation and creative visualization. The best time is in the morning when you first get up or at night before you go to bed. Create a place you can go without being interrupted. For details about how to do meditation and creative visualization, please see pages 209-213.

2. Set a time to read spiritual books or pray. In the morning or at night are both good times. For Christians, reading the Bible should be a daily routine. For others, I recommend the book *50 Spiritual Classics*, which will give you a good selection of spiritual titles to browse.

3. Create a place you can go to relax or meditate, at work and at home.

4. Find enjoyable things (people or movie, etc.) that make you laugh.

5. Write down 5 enjoyable activities and do them regularly. For example, nice soothing massage, relaxing music, a beach walk, a warm bath, etc.

Week 8
Putting It All Together

Daily Planning

An ancient Chinese proverb says: "We are born similar, but different habits set us apart." It is true that different habits make us different people. That is why we need good habits. Once an activity becomes a habit, it is easier to follow through on it more consistently.

The famous Chinese scholar, Master Zheng, said: "I review my behavior three times a day." Routinely evaluating our own behavior gives us more insight into who we are and what we are setting as our priorities. An honest evaluation will help us become better people and work more effectively.

It is a good habit to plan our daily lives and evaluate our behavior daily. Here is an example of daily planning:

List and Prioritize Daily Tasks:

1. ____________________
2. ____________________
3. ____________________
4. ____________________
5. ____________________
6. ____________________
7. ____________________
8. ____________________
9. ____________________
10. ____________________

Daily Schedule:

7:00	Exercise/reading/meditation
8:00	Breakfast
9:00	Work
10:00	
11:00	
12:00	Lunch
1:00	Break
2:00	
3:00	
4:00	
5:00	
6:00	Dinner
7:00	Relationship time
8:00	
9:00	Relaxation/exercise/reading/meditation
10:00	Bedtime

Daily review: You can develop questions to ask yourself on a daily basis.

- **What did I do today for my body?**

  — Did I eat healthy meals?
  — Did I take my supplements?
  — Did I drink eight glasses of water?
  — Did I exercise sufficiently?

- **What did I do today for my mind and spirit?**

  — Did I read the Bible or other spiritual books?
  — Did I meditate or pray?
  — Did I do something to help another person(s)?
  — Did I do something to make myself and other people laugh?
  — Did I find three things for which to be grateful?

Based on this kind of daily planning, we can also develop weekly, monthly, and yearly planning. It is a bit like planning for a trip. The more details you plan in advance, the more quickly you will arrive at your destination and the more you will enjoy your trip.

Summary

Emotional and spiritual health provides the foundation for healthy aging. This is not easy to achieve if you are suffering emotionally, or are not in touch with a purpose for your life. Healthy aging takes discipline, determination, and effort. Healthy aging is a choice and only you can decide to engage in what it takes to achieve this desirable condition.

Is it worth it?

Oh, yes.

It's you and your entire being—your vitality!

Resources

Education institutes and physician referrals:

1. Gino Tutera M.D., F.A.C.O.G.
   SottoPelle® Corporate Office
   8412 E Shea Blvd - Stc 101
   Scottsdale, AZ 85260
   Phone: 480 874-1515

   www.SottoPelletherapy.com

2. The Institute of Functional Medicine (IFM)
   4411 Pt Fosdick Drive NW - Ste 305
   Gig Harbor, WA 98335
   Phone: 800 228-0622

   www.functionalmedicine.org

3. American College for Advancement in Medicine (ACAM)
   24411 Ridge Route - Ste 115
   Laguna Hills, CA 92653
   Phone: 800 532-3688

   www.acamnet.org

4. To find a physician for pellet therapy:

   www.SottoPellelife.com

Recommended Reading

Amen, Daniel, M.D. *Change Your Brain, Change Your Life*. Three River Press, 1998.

Arpaia, Joseph, M.D. *Tibetan Wisdom for Western Life*. Beyond Words Publishing, 1999.

Butler-Bowdon, Tom. *50 Spiritual Classics: Timeless Wisdom from 50 Great Books on Inner Discovery, Enlightenment and Purpose*. Nicholas Brealey Publishing, 2005.

Caddy, Eileen. *God Spoke to Me*. Findhorn Press, 1971.

Chopra, Deepak, M.D., and David Simon. *Grow Younger, Live Longer: Ten steps to Reverse Aging*. Three Rivers Press, 2002.

Colborn Theo, Dianne Dumanoski, and John Peterson Myers. *Our Stolen Future: Are We Threatening Our Fertility, Intelligence, and Survival?—A Scientific Detective Story*. Plume, 1997.

Cornbleet, Jennifer. *Raw Food Made Easy for 1 or 2 People*. Book Publishing Company, 2005.

Dyer, Wayne, Ph.D. *10 Secrets for Success and Inner Peace*. Hay House, Inc., 2002.

Gawain, Shakti. *Creative Visualization Meditations*. New World Library, 2002.

Gittleman Ann Louise and Sears, Barry, Ph.D. *The Fat Flush Plan*. McGraw-Hill, 2002.

Hay, Louise. *You Can Heal Your Life Affirmation Kit*. 2005.

Hunt, Valerie. *Infinite Mind*. Malibu Publishing Company, 1997.

Hyman, Mark, M.D. *The UltraMind Solution: Fix Your Broken Brain By Healing Your Body First*. Scribner, 2008.

MacDonald Baker, Sidney, M.D. *Detoxification and Healing: The Key to Optimal Health*. McGraw-Hill, 2003.

Meyer, Joyce. *The Power of Simple Prayer: How to Talk with God About Everything*. The Lock Man Foundation, 2007.

Murray Michael, N.D., and Lyons, Michael. *How to Prevent and Treat Diabetes with Natural Medicine*. Riverhead Trade, 2004.

Northrup, Christiane, M.D. *The Wisdom of Menopause: Creating Physical and Emotional Health and Healing During the Change*, 2nd ed. Bantam, 2006.

Null, Gary, Ph.D. *Gary Null's Power Aging*. New American Library Trade, 2004.

Perricone, Nicholas, M.D. *The Perricone Prescription: A Physician's 28 Day Program for Total Body and Face Rejuvenation*. Collins, 2002.

Prager, Dennis. *Happiness Is a Serious Problem: A Human Nature Repair Manual*. Harper Collins, 1998.

Rogers, Sherry, M.D. *Wellness Against All Odds*. Prestige Publications, 1994.

Sears, Barry, Ph.D. *The Age-Free Zone*. Collins Living, 2000.

Shames, Richard, M.D., and Karilee Shames. *Thyroid Power: Ten Steps to Total Health*. Collins Living, 2002.

Roizen, Michael, M.D., Oz, Mehmet, M.D. *You: Staying Young: The Owner's Manual for Extending Your Warranty*. Free Press, 2007.

Somers, Suzanne. *Breakthrough: Eight Steps to Wellness*. Crown, 2008.

Sinatra, Steven, M.D. *Lower Your Blood Pressure in Eight Weeks: A Revolutionary Program for a Longer, Healthier Life*. Ballantine Books, 2003.

Sinatra, Steven, M.D., James Roberts, and Zucker, Martin. *Reverse Heart Disease Now: Stop Deadly Cardiovascular Plaque Before It's Too Late*. Wiley, 2008.

Tolle, Eckhart. *The Power of Now: A Guide To Spiritual Enlightenment*. Namaste Publishing, 1990.

Tutera, Gino, M.D. *The Real Solution to Managing Menopause and Andropause: Life Regained™*. SottoPelle® Marketing Group, Scottsdale, AZ, 2008.

Tutera, Gino, M.D. *You Don't Have to Live with It! Uncovering Nature's Power with Hormone Replacement Therapy*. SottoPelle®, Scottsdale, AZ, 2003.

Warren, Rick. *The Purpose Driven Life*. Zondervan, 2002.

Weil, Andrew, M.D. *Healthy Aging: A Lifelong Guide to Your Wellbeing*. Anchor, 2007.

Wilson, James, N.D. *Adrenal Fatigue: The 21st Century Stress Syndrome*. Smart Publications, 2002.

References

1. Ferrara A, Karter AJ, Ackerson LM, et al. Hormone replacement therapy is associate with better glycemic control in women with type 2 diabetes: The Northern California Kaiser Permanente Diabetes Registry. *Diabetes Care.* 2001;24(7):1144-1150.
2. Seely EW, Walsh BW, Gerhard MD, Williams GH. Estradiol with or without progesterone and ambulatory blood pressure in postmenopausal women. *Hypertension.* 1999;33(5):1190-1194.
3. Wagner JD. Rationale for hormone replacement in atherosclerosis prevention. *J Reprod Med.* 2000;45(3 suppl):245-258.
4. Tang MX, Jacobs D, Stern Y, et al. Effect of oestrogen during menopause on risk and age onset of Alzheimer's disease. *Lancet.* 1996;348(9025):429-432.
5. Wise PM, Dubal DB, Wilson ME, Rau SW, Böttner M. Minireview: neuroprotective effects of estrogen new insight into mechanism of action. *Endocrinology.* 2001;142(3):969-973.
6. Snow KK, Seddon JM. Age related eye diseases: impact of hormone replacement therapy, and reproductive and other risk factors. *Int J Fertil Womens Med.* 2000;45(5):301-313.
7. Writing Group for the Women's Health Initiative Investigators. Risks and benefits of estrogen plus progestin in healthy postmenopausal women: Principal results form the Women's Health Initiative randomized controlled trial. *JAMA.* 2002;288(3):321-333.
8. Yates J, Barrett-Connor E, Barlas S, Chen YT, Miller PD, Siris ES. Rapid loss of hip fracture protection after estrogen cessation: evidence from the National Osteoporosis Risk Assessment. *Obstet Gynecol.* 2004;103(3):440-446.
9. Chlebowski RT, Hendrix SL, Langer RD, et al. Influence of estrogen plus progestin on breast cancer and mammography in healthy postmenopausal women: the Women's Health Initiative randomized trial. *JAMA.* 2003;289(24):3243-3253.
10. Schairer C, Adami HO, Hoover R, Persson I. Cause specific mortality in women receiving hormone replacement therapy. *Epidemiology.* 1997;8(1):59-65.
11. Vassilopoulou –Sellin R, Asmar L, Hortobagyi GN, et al. Estrogen replacement therapy after localized breast cancer: Clinical outcome of 319 women followed prospectively. *J Clin Oncol.* 1999;17(5): 1482-1487.

12. Vassilopoulou-Sellin R, Cohen DS, Hortobagyi GN, et al. Estrogen replacement therapy for menopausal women with a history of breast carcinoma: Results of a 5 year, prospective study. *Cancer.* 2002;95(9):1817-1826.
13. Meurer LN, Lená S. Cancer recurrence and mortality in women using hormone replacement therapy after breast cancer: Meta-analysis. *J Fam Pract.* 2002;51(12):1056-1062.
14. Pasqualini JR, Gelly C, Nguyen BL, Vella C. Importance of estrogen sulfates in breast cancer. *J Steroid Biochem.* 1989;34(1-6):155-163.
15. Jefcoate CR, Liehr JC, Santen RJ, et al. Tissue-specific synthesis and oxidative metabolism of estrogens. *J Natl Cancer Inst Monogr.* 2000;27:95-112.
16. Chang M, Zhang F, Shen L, et al. Inhibition of glutathione S-transferase activity by the quinoid metabolites of equine estrogens. *Chem Res Toxicol.* 1998;11(7):758-765.
17. Chen Y, Shen L, Zhang F, et al. The equine estrogen metabolite 4-hydroxyequilenin cause DNA single-strand breaks and oxidation of DNA bases in vitro. *Chem Res Toxicol.* 1998;(11):1105-1111.
18. Cowan LD, Gordis L, Tonascia JA, Jones GS. Breast cancer incidence in women with a history of progesterone deficiency. *Am J Epidemiol.* 1981;114(2):209-217.
19. Barrat J, de Lignieres B, Marpeau L, et al. The in vivo effect of the local administration of progesterone on the mitotic activity of human ductal breast tissue. Results of a pilot study. *J Gynecol Obstet Biol Reprod.* 1990;19(3):269-274.
20. Formby B, Wiley TS. Progesterone inhibits growth and induces apoptosis in breast cancer cells: Inverse effects on Bcl-2 and p53. *Ann Clin Lab Sci.* 1998;28(6):360-369.
21. Formby B, Wiley TS. Bcl-2, survivin and variant CD44 v7-v10 are downregualted and p53 is upregulated in breast cancer cells by progesterone: Inhibition of cell growth and induction of apoptosis. *Mol Cell Biochem.* 1999;202(1-2):53-61
22. Leo JC, Wang SM, Guo CH, et al. Gene regulation profile reveals consistent anticancer properties of progesterone in hormone-independent breast cancer cells transfected with progesterone receptor. *Int J Cancer.* 2005;117(4):561-568.
23. Clarkson TB. Progesterone and cardiovascular disease. A critical review. *J Reprod Med.* 1999;44(2 suppl):180-184.
24. The writing group for the PEPI trial. Effects of estrogen or estrogen/progestin regimen on heart disease risk factors in postmenopausal women. The PEPI trial. *JAMA.* 1995;273(3):199-208.

25. Rosano GM; Webb CM, Chierchia S, et al. Natural progesterone, but not medroxyprogesterone acetate, enhances the beneficial effect of estrogen on exercise induced myocardial ischemia in postmenopausal women. *J Am Coll Cardiol.* 2000;36(7):2154-9.
26. Dimitrakakis C, Zhou J, Wang J, et al. A physiological role for testosterone in limiting estrogenic stimulation of the breast. *Menopause.* 2003;10(4):274-276.
27. Andò S, De Amicis F, Rago V, et al. Breast cancer: From estrogen to androgen receptor. *Mol Cell Endocrinol.* 2002;193(1-2):121-128.
28. Sanchez- Barcelo EJ, Cos S, Fernandz R, Mediavilla MD. Melatonin and mammary cancer: A short review. *Endocr Relat Cancer.* 2003,10(2):153-159.
29. Anisimov VN . The light-dark regimen and cancer development. *Neuro Endocrinol Lett.* 2002;Jul;23(suppl 2): 28-36.
30. Chen FP, Lee N, Soong YK, Huang KE. Comparison of transdermal and oral estrogen-replacement therapy: Effects on cardiovascular risk factors. *Menopause.* 2001;8(5):347-352.
31. Scarabin PY, Alhenc-Gelas M, Plu-Bureau G, Taisne P, Agher R, Aiach M. Effects of oral and transdermal estrogen/progesterone regimens on blood coagulation and fibrinolysis in postmenopausal women. A randomized control trial. *Artherioscler Thromb Vasc Biol.* 1997;17(11): 3071-3078.
32. Studd JW, Smith RN. Oestradiol and testosterone implants. *Baillières Clin Endocrinol Metab.* 1993;7(1):203-223.
33. Greenblatt RB, Studd JW (eds). Oestrogen therapy and the menopausal syndrome. *The Menopause. Clin Obstet Gynecol.* 1977;4(1):31-48.
34. Davelaar EM, Gerretsen G, Relyveld J. No increase in the incidence of breast carcinoma with subcutaneous administration of estradiol. *Ned Tijdschr Geneeskd.* 1991;135(14):613-615.
35. Notelovitz M, Johnston M, Smith S, Kitchens C. Metabolic and hormonal effects of 25mg and 50mg 17 beta-estradiol implants in surgically menopausal women. *Obstet Gynecol.* 1987;70(5):749-754.
36. Farrish E, Fletcher CD, Hart DM, Azzawi FA, Abdalla HI, Gray CE. The effects of hormone implants on serum lipoprotein and steroid hormones bilaterally oophorectomised women. *Acta Endocrinol (Copenh).* 1984;106(1):116-20.
37. Burger HG, Hailes J, Menelaus M, Nelson J, Hudson B, Balazs N. The management of persistent menopausal symptoms with oestradiol-testosterone implants: clinical, lipid and hormone result. *Maturitas.* 1982;6(4):351-358.

38. Studd J, Savvas M, Waston N, Garnett T, Fogelman I, Cooper D. The relationship between plasma estradiol and the increase in bone density in postmenopausal women after treatment with subcutaneous hormone implants. *Am J Obstet Gynecol.* 1990;163(5 part 1): 1474-1479.

39. Montgomery JC, Appleby L, Brincat M, et al. Effect of oestrogen and testosterone implants on psychological disorders in the climacteric. *Lancet.* 1987;1(8628):297-299.

40. Bachmann G, Bancroft J, Braunstein G, et al. Female androgen insufficiency: The Princeton consensus statement on definition, classification, and assessment. *Fertil Steril.* 2002;77(4):660-665.

41. Tutera G. *You Don't have to Live with It!* Scottsdale, AZ: SottoPelle; 2003:72.

42. Statin P, Lumme S, Tenkanen L, et al, High levels of circulating testosterone are not associated with increased prostate cancer risk: A pooled prospective study. *Int J Cancer.* 2004;108(3):418-424.

43. Rhoden EL, Morgentaler A. Testosterone replacement therapy in hypogonadal men at high risk for prostate cancer: Results of 1 year of treatment in men with prostatic intraepithelial neoplasia. *J Urol.* 2004;170(6 Pt 1);2348-2351.

44. Snyder PJ, Peachey H, Berlin JA, et al. Effects of testosterone replacement in hypogonadal men. *J Clin Endocrinol Metab.* 2000;85(8):2670-2677.

45. Cohen PG. The hypogonadal-obesity cycle: role of aromatase in modulating the testosterone-estradiol shunt—a major factor in the genesis of morbid obesity. *Med Hypotheses.* 1999;52(1):49-51.

46. Cooper MA, Ritchie EC. Testosterone replacement therapy for anxiety. *Am J Psychiatry.* 2000;157(11):1884.

47. Makinen J, Jarvisalo MJ, Pollanen P, et al. Increased carotid atherosclerosis in andropausal middle-aged men. *J Am Coll Cardiol.* 2005;45(10):1603-1608.

48. Margolese HC. The male menopause and mood: Testosterone decline and depression in the aging male—Is there a link? *J Geriatr Psychiatry Neurol.* 2000;13(2):93-101.

49. Hak AE, Witteman JC, de Jong FH, Geerlings MI, Hofman A, Pols HA. Low levels of endogenous androgens increase the risk of atherosclerosis in elderly men: The Rotterdam Study. *J Clin Endocrinol Metab.* 2002;87(8):3632-3639.

50. Wang C, Swerdloff RS, Iranmanesh A, et al. Testosterone improves sexual function, mood, and muscle strength and body composition parameters in hypogonadal men. *J Clin Endocrinol Metab.* 2000;85(8):2839-2853.

51. Rosano G, Leonardo F, Pagnotta P, et al. Acute anti-ischemic effect of testosterone in men with coronary artery disease. *Circulation.* 1999;99(13):1666-1670.
52. Stellato RK, Feldman HA, Hamdy O, Horton ES, McKinlay JB. Testosterone, sex hormone-binding globulin, and the development of type 2 diabetes in middle-aged men: prospective results from the Massachusetts male aging study. *Diabetes Care*. 2000;23(4):490-494.
53. Dhindsa S, Prabhakar S, Sethi M, Bandyopadhyay A, Chaudhuri A, Dandona P. Frequent occurrence of hypogonadotropic hypogonadism in type II diabetes. *J Clin Endocrinol Metab.* 2004;89:5462-5468.
54. Moffat SD, Zonderman AB, Metter EJ, Blackman MR, Harman SM, Resnick SM. Longitudinal assessment of serum free testosterone concentration predicts memory performance and cognitive status in elderly men. *J Clin Endocrinol Metab*. 2002;87(11):5001-5007.
55. Gouras GK, Xu H, Gross RS, et al. Testosterone reduces neuronal secretion of Alzheimer's beta amyloid peptides. *Proc Natl Acad Sci USA*. 2000;97(3):1202-1205.
56. Eastell R, Boyle IT, Compston J, et al. Management of male osteoporosis: report of the UK Consensus group. *QJM*. 1998;91(2):71-92.
57. AACE Thyroid Task Force. American Association of Clinical Endocrinologists medical guidelines for clinical practice for the evaluation and treatment of hyperthyroidism and hypothyroidism. *Endocr Pract.* 2002;8(6):457-469.
58. Brucker DF. Effects of environmental synthetic chemicals on the thyroid function. *Thyroid.* 1998;8(9):827-856.
59. Colquhoun J. Why I changed my mind about water fluoridation. *Perspect Biol Med.* 1997;41(1):29-44.
60. Baisier WV, Hertoghe J, W. Eeckhaut W. Thyroid insufficiency. Is thyroxine the only valuable drug? *J Nutr Environ Med.* 2001;11(3):159-166.
61. Levin HS, Rodnitzky RL. Behavioral effects of organophosphate pesticides in man. *Clin Tox.* 1976;9(3):391-405.
62. Feldman RG, Ricks NL, Baker EL, Neuropsychological effects of industrial toxins: A review. *Am J Ind Med.* 1980;1(2):211-227.
63. White R, Jobling S, Hoare SA, Sumpter JP, Parker MG, et al. Environmentally persistent alkylphenolic compounds are estrogenic. *Endocrinology.* 1994;135(1):175-182.
64. Shenker BJ, TL Guo TL, Shapiro IM. Low level methylmercury exposure causes human T cells to undergo apoptosis: evidence of mitochondrial dysfunction. *Environ Res.* 1998;77:149-59.

65. DeSouza Queiroz ML, Pena SC, Salles TSI, de Capitani EM, Olalla Saad ST. Abnormal antioxidant system in erythrocytes of mercury exposed workers. *Human & Exp Toxicol.* 1998;17:225-230.

66. Ngim CH, Foo SC, Boey KW, JeyaratnamJ. Chronic neurobehavioral effects of elemental mercury in dentists. *Brit J Indust Med.* 1992;49:782-790.

67. Solonen JT, Seppänen K, Nyyssönen K, et al. Intake of mercury from fish, lipid peroxidation, and the risk of myocardial infarction and coronary, cardiovascular, and early death in eastern Finnish men. *Circulation.* 1995;91(3):645-655.

68. Perl DP, Brody AR. Alzheimer's disease: X-ray spectrometric evidence of aluminum accumulation in neurofibrillary tangle-bearing neurons. *Sci.* 1980;208(4441):297-299.

69. Folsom AR, Aleksic N, Catellier D, et al. C-reactive protein and incident coronary heart disease in the atherosclerosis risk in communities (ARIC) study. *Am Heart J.* 2002;144(2):233-238.

70. Futterman LG, Lemberg L. High-sensitive C-reactive protein is the most effective prognostic measurement of acute coronary events. *Am J Crit Care.* 2002;11(5):482-486.

71. Clarke, R, Daly L, Robinson K, et al. Hyperhomocysteine: An independent factor for vascular disease. *N Eng J Med,* 1991;324:1149-1155.

72. Motoyama T, Sano H, Fukuzaki H. Oral magnesium supplementation in patients with essential hypertension. *Hypertension.* 1989;13:227-232.

73. Cantor KP, Lynch CF, Hildesheim ME, et al. Drinking water source and chlorination by-products. I. Risk of bladder cancer. *Epidemiology.* 1998;9:21-28.

74. Porta M, Malats N, Jariod M, et al. Serum concentration of organochlorine compounds and K-ras mutations in exocrine pancreatic cancer. PANKRAS II Study Group. *Lancet.* 1999;354(9196):2125-2130.

75. DeFronzo RA, Ferranni E. Insulin resistance: A multifaceted syndrome responsible for NIDDM, obesity, hypertension, dyslipidemia, and atherosclerotic cardiovascular disease. *Diabetes Care.* 1991:14(3):173-194.

Index